the omega solution

Fix Your Fats, Fuel Your Future

the 100+living plan
book five

Dr Graham Jenkins BSc DC

contents

the omega solution: fix your fats, fuel your future

The Fat Dilemma

When Sarah first walked into my office, she looked like the picture of modern life – harried, overworked, and exhausted. At 42, she was juggling a demanding corporate career, raising two teenagers, and caring for her aging mother. The weight of it all was visible in her slumped posture, her tired eyes, and the way she sighed before she even sat down.

"I don't even know where to start," she said, dropping her bag beside the chair. "I'm tired all the time. I can't focus. My joints ache, my skin looks terrible, and I swear I'm aging faster than ever. I'm doing the best I can, but life is... well, you know."

I nodded. Sarah's story was all too familiar. She was one of many patients I've seen over the past 30 years who had fallen into the trap of modern living: too busy to cook, too tired to exercise, and too stressed to think clearly. Her diet, like so many others, had devolved into whatever was most convenient – processed foods and a steady stream of takeout.

"What do you eat in a typical day?" I asked.

Sarah winced. "Honestly? Coffee for breakfast, maybe a muffin if I have time. Lunch is usually something quick, like a sandwich or salad from the deli in my office building. And dinner... well, I'm so tired by the end of the day that we usually have something delivered – pizza, Chinese, whatever the kids want."

She paused. "I know it's not good for me. I just don't have the time or energy to figure out something better. And it feels like I'm paying for it."

Sarah wasn't wrong. Her body was paying for it. She was stuck in the Standard American Diet (SAD) cycle – a diet packed with ultra processed foods and seed oils, overloaded with omega-6 fats and severely lacking in omega-3s. This imbalance was wreaking havoc on her energy, her mood, her joints, and even her skin.

The ultra-processed foods were just empty calories, offering her body nothing to build on. Even though she maintained a reasonably "healthy" weight, her body was breaking down from the inside out, and none of the essential building blocks were there for her cells to rebuild any reasonable form of health.

What Sarah didn't realize was how much of her fatigue, brain fog, and chronic aches were tied to her imbalance of fats. It wasn't just about what she wasn't eating – like vegetables or lean proteins – it was about the harmful fats she was consuming in excess. And she wasn't alone.

The reality is that most North Americans are living with this hidden imbalance. Our modern diets have tipped the scales dramatically toward omega-6 fatty acids, mostly from ultra-processed foods and vegetable oils, while omega-3 – the fat that supports cellular health, reduces inflammation, and protect against aging – has become a rare guest at the table.

It's no wonder Sarah felt like she was falling apart.

This is where the omega-3/omega-6 balance comes in. It's the missing piece in many of our health puzzles, quietly affecting everything from our brains to our hearts, our joints to our skin. When we fix this balance, we begin to restore our bodies to their natural state of health and vitality.

Sarah's Journey Begins

With a sigh of relief, Sarah agreed to take the first steps toward change. It didn't happen overnight, but with small, manageable adjustments –

replacing processed foods with whole, nutrient-dense ones, adding omega-3 rich foods into her meals, and learning to identify hidden omega-6s – Sarah began to feel the difference. Her energy improved, her mood lifted, and her joint pain eased. Over time, her brain fog cleared, her skin glowed, and for the first time in years, she felt like herself again.

She was slowly adopting a lifestyle that built health and vitality. For Sarah, this was one of the key elements in her 100+Living Plan. A plan that I have used with thousands of families to help regain their health, revive their joy and start pointing their life towards longevity.

This book is built around Sarah's story because her journey is one so many of us share. It's a journey of discovering the power of omega-3s and how, by fixing the fats in our diets, we can fuel our future with better health, more vitality, and a longer life.

Why This Book Matters: The Omega Solution for Longevity and Health

As I've seen time and time again in my practice, the real turning point in health isn't always some massive overhaul or radical lifestyle change. Often, it's the small, intentional shifts that make the biggest difference. This is especially true when it comes to the fats we consume. Our modern diet has gone off course, and the imbalance of omega-3 and omega-6 fatty acids is quietly stealing our vitality, contributing to chronic inflammation, and accelerating the aging process.

Why does this matter so much? Because fats are not just fuel – they are the very building blocks of our cells. They form the membranes that protect our cells, fuel our brains, reduce inflammation, and keep our hearts beating strong. When we neglect the right fats – specifically omega-3s – we neglect the very essence of our health.

There's a quote I often think of from Dr. Andrew Weil, a pioneer in integrative medicine, that perfectly captures this: "The single most important dietary change you can make to reduce inflammation is to increase your intake of omega-3 fatty acids and decrease your intake of omega-6 fatty acids." This simple shift can change the entire trajectory of your health, and yet, so few people realize it.

When you begin to understand how crucial this fat balance is, the pieces start to fall into place. It's not just about avoiding disease – it's about thriving in every area of life. Omega-3s have been shown to support everything from brain function to heart health, from reducing the risk of neurodegenerative diseases to improving mood and mental clarity. It's about living with the kind of vitality that not only keeps you going longer but keeps you feeling better for years to come.

One of the reasons I wrote this book is because, like my patient Sarah, many people simply don't realize how impactful these fats are. They come into my office feeling sluggish, inflamed, and disconnected from their own bodies, and they can't understand why. The truth is, they're often stuck in what I call the "fat trap" – consuming too many omega-6 fats from processed and fast foods, and not nearly enough omega-3s. It's a silent epidemic, and it's robbing us of our longevity and health.

Dr. Mark Hyman, another leader in functional medicine, said it well, "Omega-3 fats are like the oil that keeps your engine running smoothly. Without enough, your engine is going to break down over time." This breakdown isn't just something that happens when we're older. It begins earlier than most of us think, slowly affecting our cells, our cognitive function, and our immune system.

This book is about fixing that. "The Omega Solution" offers a roadmap to reclaiming your health by understanding the fats you eat and making intentional choices that serve your long-term well-being. You don't have to settle for feeling 'just okay' or 'getting by' day after day. By balancing your omega-3 and omega-6 intake, you can unlock a level of health that allows you to enjoy life at its fullest.

Whether you're already on a journey to improve your health or you're just starting out, this book is designed to empower you with practical steps and the science behind them. It's about offering hope and possibility – that with the right knowledge, you can take control of your health, live longer, and feel better than you ever thought possible.

Together, we'll explore how fixing your fats can fuel your future, adding years to your life and life to your years. Because as I often tell my patients: "It's not just about living longer – it's about living better." And the omega-3 solution, for many, is where that journey begins.

Our Modern Diet: The Problem with Seed Oils and Processed Fats

When we take a closer look at the way most of us eat today, it's easy to see where things went off the rails. The convenience of modern life has brought with it a reliance on ultra processed foods – meals that are quick, cheap, and, unfortunately, filled with unhealthy fats. One of the biggest culprits? Seed oils.

These oils – found in everything from salad dressings to fast food – are incredibly high in omega-6 fatty acids. And while omega-6 fats aren't inherently bad (in fact, we need them in small amounts), the problem lies in the overwhelming imbalance they create when consumed in excess. In the past, our diets had a natural balance of omega-3 to omega-6. But today, the typical ratio has been thrown out of whack, with most of us consuming 15 to 20 times more omega-6 than omega-3. This imbalance fuels inflammation, contributes to chronic disease, and accelerates aging.

Dr. Cate Shanahan, a leading expert on nutrition, sums it up well, "Vegetable oils are the worst ingredients in our food supply, and if you removed them, you would completely eliminate many of the most common diseases in North America." These seed oils – like soybean, corn, and sunflower oil – are everywhere in our food supply, often hidden in products we don't even think of as unhealthy.

Processed foods, packed with these oils, have become the backbone of the Standard American Diet (SAD). I've seen the effects of this diet firsthand. Patients come to me wondering why they feel sluggish, why their joints ache, or why they're gaining weight despite eating what they believe is a "normal" diet. It's frustrating because they don't realize that so much of what they're eating is engineered to be cheap and shelf-stable, not nutritious.

Dr. David Ludwig, a professor of nutrition at Harvard, puts it like this, "Processed foods, full of refined carbohydrates and unhealthy fats, disrupt our metabolism, promote inflammation, and accelerate aging." It's not about calories; it's about the quality of the food we're consuming. And when we rely on processed foods loaded with seed oils, we're setting ourselves up for a lifetime of poor health outcomes.

But here's the good news – we can change this. The body is resilient, and by making small, manageable shifts in the way we eat, we can correct the damage done by years of consuming the wrong fats. The goal isn't perfection; it's about creating balance.

The omega-3/omega-6 ratio isn't just a trendy concept – it's a fundamental shift in how we approach our health. When we start prioritizing omega-3-rich foods like fatty fish, flaxseeds, and walnuts while cutting back on omega-6-laden processed foods, we can begin to tip the scales back in our favor. The best part? These changes don't just improve how we feel in the short term – they set the stage for a longer, healthier life.

This book is your guide to understanding how those tiny decisions – like what oil you cook with or what snacks you choose – can either support or undermine your health. You don't have to overhaul your entire diet overnight. But by understanding the problem with seed oils and processed fats, and by taking steps to fix your fat intake, you'll be well on your way to reclaiming your vitality.

As Dr. Mark Hyman often says, "Food is information – it talks to your genes, it tells them what to do. And when you eat the right fats, you send the right messages to your body." That's the hope behind this book – that with the right information, you can make empowered choices that fuel not just your body, but your future.

So, let's get started. We're going to explore how the fats you eat can make all the difference in your energy, your health, and your longevity. It's time to fix your fats and fuel your future.

one
the omega imbalance – how we (and sarah) got here

WHEN SARAH first walked into my office, she was a living example of what's happened to so many of us in today's world – overwhelmed, stressed, and unknowingly trapped in a cycle of poor nutrition. It wasn't that she didn't care about her health; in fact, she desperately wanted to feel better. But between the demands of her job and family, she had little time to think about what she was putting into her body. Like many of us, Sarah had fallen victim to the convenience of fast food, takeout, and processed meals.

"I just don't have time to cook healthy meals," she told me, reflecting the struggle so many people face. When life gets hectic, nutrition is often the first thing to fall by the wayside. Processed foods – quick, easy, and marketed as harmless – become the go-to.

What Sarah didn't realize, though, was that this "easy" way of eating was contributing to her fatigue, inflammation, and lack of mental clarity. The problem wasn't just that she wasn't eating enough fresh, whole foods; it was the type of fats she was consuming. She was caught in the "fat trap". Her diet was overloaded with omega-6 fatty acids from ultra processed oils and sorely lacking in omega-3s. The result? A perfect storm for inflammation, sluggishness, and premature aging.

How did we get here? How did Sarah – and the rest of us – end up so far off course?

Historical Perspective on Fats: From Whole Foods to Processed Oils

To understand the omega-3/omega-6 imbalance in our modern diet, we need to take a step back and look at how fats have evolved – or rather, devolved – over time. Not too long ago, people consumed fats primarily from whole, unprocessed foods. Traditional diets included things like fatty fish, nuts, seeds, and even animal fats from pasture-raised animals. These sources were naturally rich in omega-3s, and the balance of omega-3 to omega-6 in the diet was much closer to what our bodies are designed for.

But with the rise of industrial food production in the 20th century, everything changed. Whole foods were replaced by ultra processed ones, and naturally occurring fats gave way to cheaper, industrial seed oils like soybean, corn, and sunflower oil and might I add, all crops that have been heavily subsidized with your tax dollars on behalf of the food processing industry. These oils are not only heavily processed but also extremely high in omega-6 fatty acids, which throw off the delicate balance our bodies need.

It wasn't just the oils that changed – it was the entire landscape of our food. The government and food industries started pushing the idea that low-fat, high carb diets were the key to good health, demonizing natural fats like butter and coconut oil in favor of processed, fat-free foods. And the worst part? This shift was driven not by sound science, but by manipulated studies funded by food corporations.

Dr. Robert Lustig, a pediatric endocrinologist and a leading voice on nutrition, has been vocal about this. He says, "The fact is, processed food is not real food. It's not food anymore; it's a food-like substance." And nowhere is this truer than with the oils we consume.

The food pyramid that so many of us grew up with reinforced this misguided message. We were told to avoid fats, load up on carbohydrates, and trust in ultra processed, low-fat options. But the truth is, the pyramid wasn't built on sound nutritional advice. It was shaped, in large part, by industries with vested interests. As an example, even though high-fructose corn syrup – a concoction with no business being in the human body – was pushed as a safe sweetener, we now know the devastating effects it has on metabolic health and skyrocketing rates of type 2 diabetes.

And fats are no different. Ultra processed oils, supported by manipulated studies, have made their way into the majority of our packaged foods, leaving the consumer confused and misled. These oils are now a staple in the Standard American Diet (SAD), and we are paying the price with rising rates of chronic disease, inflammation, and poor health outcomes.

Nutrition expert and author Nina Teicholz puts it bluntly, "For decades, we have been told to eat less fat, but it turns out that's not just bad advice, it's wrong. The science never supported it. We've been led astray by flawed studies and the influence of powerful industries."

The irony is that the very fats we've been taught to avoid – omega-3-rich fats from fish, flaxseeds, and healthy oils like olive oil – are the ones our bodies are craving. Meanwhile, the fats we've been consuming in abundance – those found in ultra processed oils – are driving inflammation and disease. This is where the imbalance begins, and why so many, like Sarah, find themselves stuck in a cycle of poor health without even realizing it.

The good news? It's never too late to change. By returning to a diet that prioritizes whole, nutrient-rich fats and restores the balance between omega-3 and omega-6, we can reverse the damage done by years of poor dietary advice. As Dr. Catherine Shanahan, a leading authority on nutrition and genetics, has said, "The human body is incredibly resilient. When you start feeding it real food, it knows what to do with it."

And that's the key: getting back to real food and healthy fats, ones that support your body's natural ability to thrive. So, how did we get here? Through decades of bad advice, ultra processed foods, and industrial seed oils. But with the right information – and the right fats – we can get back on track, just like Sarah.

This book is about showing you how.

The Standard American Diet (SAD): The Rise of Omega-6

Let's be honest: the Standard American Diet (SAD) is aptly named. It's not just an unfortunate acronym – it's a reflection of the state of our health. The SAD is a dietary landscape that's become completely unbalanced, driven by convenience, cost, and profit rather than what's best for our bodies. One of the biggest casualties in this shift has been our relationship with fats, particularly the balance between omega-6 and omega-3 fatty acids.

Over the years, I've seen firsthand how people like Sarah get trapped in the cycle of fast food, processed meals, and snacks that are often marketed as healthy. These foods are loaded with omega-6 fats, primarily from seed oils like corn, soybean, and sunflower oil. They're cheap, shelf-stable, and heavily used by the food industry to mass-produce nearly everything you see in the middle aisles of the grocery store.

It wasn't always this way. Decades ago, our diets were much more balanced. We consumed omega-3s from fatty fish, grass-fed meats, and plants like flax and chia seeds. Omega-6s were still present, but they came from natural sources like nuts and seeds – and in moderation. But as the industrial food system took over, that balance was thrown out of whack.

Today, the average American is consuming an omega-6 to omega-3 ratio of anywhere from 15:1 to 20:1. That's a far cry from the ideal ratio of 1:1 or even 2:1, which is closer to what our ancestors ate. This imbalance is at the heart of so many modern health issues – chronic inflammation, heart disease, obesity, and even mental health disorders.

Dr. Artemis Simopoulos, a leading expert on omega-3 and omega-6 fatty acids, has been sounding the alarm for years. She said, "Our ancestors evolved on a diet with a ratio of omega-6 to omega-3 essential fatty acids of about 1:1, whereas in Western diets the ratio is 15:1 to 16.7:1. Such a high omega-6/omega-3 ratio promotes the pathogenesis of many diseases, including cardiovascular disease, cancer, and inflammatory and autoimmune diseases."

It's not just about eating too much omega-6 – it's about the absence of omega-3s to balance it out. Omega-6s, in moderation, play a role in the body's inflammatory response, which is necessary for healing. But when omega-6s are consumed in excess, as they are in the Standard American Diet, that inflammatory response becomes chronic. And chronic inflammation is at the root of so many diseases we face today.

So, how did omega-6 fats become so dominant? It all comes down to the food industry's shift toward processed oils in the 20th century. Seed oils like soybean, corn, and cottonseed oil became the backbone of processed foods because they were cheap to produce and had a long shelf life. These oils were embraced by the food industry and marketed as a healthier alternative to saturated fats. And because they were so cost-effective, they quickly found their way into almost every packaged food product on the market.

Dr. Joseph Hibbeln, a clinical investigator who has done extensive research on omega-3 and omega-6 fats, explains it this way, "The increased use of seed oils, which are high in omega-6 fatty acids, parallels the rise in chronic diseases, particularly inflammatory diseases. These oils are pervasive in the food system and are directly contributing to the imbalanced omega-6 to omega-3 ratio."

Let's not forget the role the government played in this shift. For years, we were told to avoid fats – particularly saturated fats – based on flawed research that vilified them as the root of heart disease. This gave rise to the low-fat craze of the 1980s and 1990s, during which we were all encouraged to eat more carbohydrates and avoid fat like the plague. But in the absence of fats, what did the food industry do? It replaced them with sugar, refined carbohydrates, and those ubiquitous seed oils.

As Dr. David Perlmutter, neurologist and author, puts I,: "The low-fat, high-carbohydrate advice that has dominated our dietary recommendations for decades has contributed to the very diseases it was meant to prevent. And the fats we have been consuming – like omega-6s from processed oils – are making the situation even worse."

And here we are today, with a diet that's not just deficient in essential nutrients but actively contributing to our health problems. The SAD has become a breeding ground for inflammation and disease. The convenience of fast food and processed snacks is coming at a cost that's too high to ignore.

Dr. Michael Crawford, a renowned expert on the role of fats in human development, said, "The human brain is uniquely dependent on omega-3 fatty acids. If we want to maintain cognitive function and prevent diseases like Alzheimer's, we need to rethink the fats we're eating."

By rethinking the fats we're eating, restoring the balance between omega-3 and omega-6, and reclaiming our health. The rise of omega-6 in the Standard American Diet doesn't have to be a permanent fixture in your life. With the right information and the right choices, we can shift the balance, reduce inflammation, and set ourselves on a path to better health.

The key is understanding that what we eat today shapes our health tomorrow. By prioritizing omega-3-rich foods and reducing our intake of ultra processed, omega-6-heavy oils, we can make a meaningful difference in our longevity, mental clarity, and overall well-being.

It will take a new way of thinking to fix this imbalance but the results are worth every step. My goal with this book is to encourage you that this change is easier than you think and far more rewarding that you will ever know. You've got this.

Omega-3 vs. Omega-6: Why the Ratio Matters for Your Health

Let's break down why this ratio of omega-3 to omega-6 fats is so critical for your health. At first glance, it might seem like a technical detail, but the balance between these two essential fatty acids holds the key to many of the health problems we face today.

Both omega-3 and omega-6 fats are polyunsaturated fatty acids, and they're called "essential" because our bodies can't produce them. We have to get them from our diet. While both play important roles in our biology, they have very different effects on our health, especially when it comes to inflammation.

Omega-6 fats, as we previously mentioned are commonly found in seed oils like soybean, corn, and sunflower oil, are pro-inflammatory. Now, before we vilify them completely, it's important to recognize that inflammation isn't always bad. In fact, inflammation is a necessary part of our immune response. It's what helps us heal from injuries and fight off infections. However, when omega-6 intake becomes excessive – as it does in the Standard American Diet (SAD) – it promotes chronic inflammation, which is a root cause of many diseases, from heart disease to cancer.

On the other hand, omega-3 fats, which are found in foods like fatty fish, flaxseeds, and walnuts, are anti-inflammatory. These fats help keep inflammation in check, support brain function, and promote heart health. They also play a critical role in cell membrane integrity and the regulation of gene expression.

Here's where the ratio comes into play: For optimal health, we need a balance between omega-3s and omega-6s. The ideal ratio is somewhere around 1:1 or 2:1, meaning for every gram of omega-6 you consume, you should be getting at least an equal amount, if not slightly more, omega-3s. However, in the modern diet, this ratio has been pushed to a staggering 15:1 or even 20:1 in favor of omega-6s. That's a huge imbalance, and it's wreaking havoc on our health.

Dr. Bill Lands, a prominent biochemist and researcher in lipid (fat) metabolism, explains it well, "When the omega-6 and omega-3 balance shifts too far toward omega-6, it amplifies inflammatory responses in the body and increases the risk of many chronic diseases. A diet with a proper balance can suppress inflammation and improve overall health."

So, why does this matter so much? When we consistently consume too many omega-6 fats without balancing them with enough omega-3s, our bodies become predisposed to chronic inflammation. And chronic inflammation is like a slow burn – it's not something you notice right away, but over time, it starts to damage tissues, leading to issues like heart disease, arthritis, diabetes, and even neurological disorders.

Omega-3s, especially EPA (eicosapentaenoic acid) and DHA (docosahexaenoic acid), which are found in fish like salmon and mackerel, counteract this inflammation. They help regulate the production of inflammatory molecules in the body, acting as a natural brake on inflammation. That's why diets high in omega-3s are associated with lower risks of heart disease, better brain health, and even improved mood and cognitive function.

Dr. Jeffrey Bland, a leader in functional medicine, summarizes the importance of this balance, "The relationship between omega-3 and omega-6 fats is one of the most important dietary balances we need to pay attention to. It's not about avoiding fats; it's about choosing the right ones in the right proportions. When we get this balance wrong, inflammation runs rampant, but when we correct it, we can dramatically improve our health."

What's fascinating is that omega-3 and omega-6 fats compete for the same enzymes in the body – the enzymes that convert these fats into signaling molecules like prostaglandins, thromboxanes, and leukotrienes. These molecules either promote or reduce inflammation. When your diet is overloaded with omega-6s, they dominate the enzyme pathways, leading to the production of pro-inflammatory molecules. But when omega-3s are present in sufficient quantities, they occupy those same pathways and produce anti-inflammatory molecules instead.

It's like a tug of war happening inside your body – omega-6s pulling toward inflammation and omega-3s pulling toward anti-inflammation. If you're not eating enough omega-3s, your body is stuck in a pro-inflammatory state, and that chronic inflammation sets the stage for disease.

Dr. Michael Murray, a naturopathic physician and author on nutrition, notes, "We have ample evidence that the balance of omega-3 and omega-6 fats in the diet can influence everything from cardiovascular health to mental well-being. When we restore that balance, we give our bodies the chance to heal, to reduce inflammation, and to thrive."

So, what can we do? The good news is that this imbalance is something we can fix with intentional changes to our diet. By reducing the intake of omega-6-rich ultra processed foods and seed oils and increasing our consumption of omega-3-rich foods like fatty fish, chia seeds, and flaxseeds, we can start to restore the balance. And when we restore that balance, the results can be transformative: less inflammation, more energy, improved cognitive function, and better long-term health.

The ratio of omega-3 to omega-6 might seem like a small detail, but it's a powerful determinant of your overall health. It's not about cutting out fats – it's about understanding which fats serve your body best and how to create the balance that will support longevity, vitality, and well-being.

In the end, fixing your fats is one of the most important steps you can take toward a healthier, more vibrant life. By addressing the omega-3/omega-6 ratio, we're not just treating symptoms – we're going after the root cause of chronic inflammation, giving your body the tools it needs to thrive.

two
omega-3s and longevity – the key to a long, healthy life

Sarah's Guilt and the Hope for Change

AS SARAH SAT across from me in the office, she shifted uncomfortably in her chair, her voice barely above a whisper. "I just feel like I'm failing them," she admitted, her eyes welling up with tears. "I want to do better for my kids, for myself, but there's no time. Between work, soccer practices, and just trying to keep everything from falling apart, the only thing I can manage is ordering takeout. And I know... I know it's not good for them."

Her guilt was palpable, and it's a feeling I've seen too many times to count. In a world where the demands on our time are constantly increasing, it's so easy to feel like we're falling short, especially when it comes to feeding ourselves and our families. Sarah's story isn't just her own – it's the story of so many parents and individuals who are trying to keep up with life's pace, only to find that their health and the health of their loved ones is slipping through their fingers.

The irony is that Sarah, like so many others, wants to do better. She wants to provide nourishing, healthy meals for her teenagers, to model good habits, and to feel better in her own skin. But between the daily grind and the constant barrage of unhealthy options, it can feel impossible.

I reminded Sarah of that she wasn't stuck in this rut forever. With just a few small adjustments, we could start turning things around, not just for her but for her family too. The beauty of nutrition is that it doesn't have to be perfect to have a positive impact. And when we start with something as simple – and powerful – as omega-3s, we can set the foundation for a lifetime of better health, for ourselves and for the ones we love.

Sarah's journey toward health wasn't about radical change or an overhaul of her lifestyle. It was about small, manageable steps, starting with understanding the power of omega-3s and how they could help her family regain their vitality. And this is where her story, and perhaps yours, begins to shift.

The Science of Longevity: How Omega-3s Protect Cells

When we talk about longevity – living a long, healthy life – we have to start at the cellular level. After all, your cells are the building blocks of everything that happens in your body. And if your cells aren't functioning properly, neither are you. This is where omega-3 fatty acids come in. These fats aren't just good for you – they're essential for protecting your cells and promoting longevity.

At the heart of it, omega-3s help to maintain the structure and function of cell membranes. Your cell membranes act like the gatekeepers of your cells, controlling what comes in and what goes out. When your cell membranes are healthy, your cells can communicate better, process nutrients more efficiently, and fend off damage from harmful substances. Omega-3s, particularly the EPA (eicosapentaenoic acid) and DHA (docosahexaenoic acid) forms, integrate into these cell membranes, keeping them flexible and resilient.

Dr. William Harris, a renowned researcher in omega-3s and cardiovascular health, has described it well, "When omega-3s are incorporated into cell membranes, they make the membranes more fluid and flexible. This improves cell function, helps reduce inflammation, and promotes better overall health."

But the benefits go even deeper. Omega-3s also play a crucial role in reducing oxidative stress – one of the key factors in aging. Oxidative stress occurs when harmful molecules called free radicals damage your cells, accelerating the aging process and contributing to chronic diseases. Omega-3s act like a shield, protecting your cells from this oxidative damage and helping to neutralize free radicals.

It's also important to mention that omega-3s support mitochondrial function. Mitochondria are the energy powerhouses of your cells, responsible for producing the energy your body needs to function. When your mitochondria are healthy and operating efficiently, your cells have the energy they need to repair themselves, fight off disease, and keep you feeling vibrant. Studies have shown that omega-3s help improve mitochondrial function, which translates to better energy production and cellular repair.

Dr. Rhonda Patrick, a leading expert in longevity research has said, "Omega-3 fatty acids not only reduce inflammation but also help maintain mitochondrial function and support cellular energy production. This has profound implications for aging and disease prevention."

One of the most exciting aspects of omega-3 research is its potential role in slowing telomere shortening. Telomeres are the protective caps at the ends of your chromosomes, and as you age, they naturally shorten. Shorter telomeres are associated with aging and an increased risk of chronic diseases. But here's the good news: research has shown that higher omega-3 levels are associated with slower telomere shortening, which could mean a slower aging process at the cellular level.

Dr. Elizabeth Blackburn, a Nobel Prize-winning scientist known for her work on telomeres, stated "Omega-3s appear to play a protective role in slowing the biological aging process by reducing the rate of telomere shortening."

So, when we talk about omega-3s and longevity, we're talking about more than just adding years to your life. We're talking about adding healthy years – years where your cells are functioning optimally, your body is resilient, and your mind stays sharp.

For Sarah, understanding how omega-3s could protect her cells and slow down the aging process was a game-changer. It wasn't just about what she ate today – it was about the long-term impact those choices would have on her health and her family's well-being. By incorporating more omega-3s into their diet, she could start laying the foundation for a future filled with vitality, not just for herself, but for her kids as well.

And as I continue to mention, it doesn't take an extreme diet or a complete lifestyle overhaul to start reaping the benefits of omega-3s. Small changes, like adding more omega-3-rich foods to your meals or taking a high-quality omega-3 supplement, can make a big difference. The science is clear – omega-3s protect your cells, reduce inflammation, and promote longevity. And with every bite, you're giving your body the tools it needs to thrive, now and for years to come.

Inflammation and Aging: Omega-3s as the Natural Anti-inflammatory

If there's one thing I've learned in my years of practice, it's that inflammation is a part of almost every chronic condition that walks through my door. From heart disease to joint pain, fatigue to cognitive decline, inflammation plays a major role in how our bodies break down over time. What many people don't realize, though, is that inflammation is also a key driver of aging itself.

We often think of aging as something that just happens, a natural process we can't do anything about. But the truth is, how we age – and how quickly – is deeply tied to chronic inflammation. When inflammation is left unchecked, it accelerates the wear and tear on your body, leading to what researchers now call "inflammaging." The good news? Omega-3s are one of the most powerful natural tools we have to fight back against this process.

Inflammation is your body's way of protecting itself when something's wrong. If you cut yourself or catch a cold, inflammation is a natural and necessary part of the healing process. The problem arises when inflammation becomes chronic – when your body's immune system is constantly on high alert, even when there's no real threat. That's what happens when your diet is overloaded with processed foods, sugar, and omega-6 fats, and it leads to long-term damage.

Dr. Barry Sears, creator of the Zone Diet and a pioneer in the field of inflammation research, sums it up perfectly, "Inflammation is the underlying cause of chronic disease. Control the inflammation, and you can control the disease process."

This is where omega-3s come in as the body's natural anti-inflammatory. Omega-3 fatty acids, particularly EPA and DHA, help reduce inflammation by competing with omega-6s for the same enzymes. While omega-6s promote the production of pro-inflammatory molecules, omega-3s shift the balance in favor of anti-inflammatory molecules. They calm the immune response, keeping inflammation in check and protecting your cells from unnecessary damage.

When you eat a diet rich in omega-3s, you're essentially giving your body the tools it needs to dial down the inflammation. This has far-reaching effects, not only in reducing the risk of chronic diseases but also in slowing the aging process itself. Chronic inflammation wears away at your tissues, leads to the degradation of collagen (which keeps your skin and joints healthy), and accelerates the decline of your cells. By reducing inflammation, omega-3s help protect these structures, allowing your body to age more gracefully.

Dr. Nicholas Perricone, a dermatologist and anti-aging expert, is a big proponent of omega-3s for this very reason. He says, "Omega-3 fatty acids are the most powerful anti-inflammatory nutrients. They not only reduce inflammation in the body but also in the skin, leading to better overall health and a more youthful appearance."

It's also important to recognize the role that inflammation plays in some of the most serious age-related diseases. For example, chronic inflammation is closely linked to heart disease, which remains the leading cause of death in the world. Omega-3s have been shown to reduce markers of inflammation, like C-reactive protein (CRP), which is a strong predictor of heart disease. By lowering inflammation, omega-3s help protect your cardiovascular system, reducing the risk of heart attacks and strokes.

In the brain, inflammation plays a role in neurodegenerative diseases like Alzheimer's and dementia. Over time, unchecked inflammation can damage neurons, leading to cognitive decline. But omega-3s, particularly DHA, are known to have neuroprotective effects, reducing inflammation in the brain and supporting cognitive function.

Dr. Michael Greger, a well-known physician and author, puts it this way, "Omega-3 fatty acids have anti-inflammatory properties that protect our arteries and our brains. They're nature's defense system against chronic inflammation, which is a key driver of aging and disease."

For Sarah, learning about inflammation and how it was impacting her body was a turning point. The joint pain, the fatigue, the brain fog – they all had roots in chronic inflammation, driven by years of processed foods and a lack of omega-3s in her diet. But the moment she started to shift that balance by incorporating more omega-3-rich foods, she began to notice changes. Her energy levels improved, her joints felt better, and even her skin started to look more vibrant. It wasn't just about feeling better in the short term – it was about building a foundation for a healthier, more resilient future.

And this is the hopeful part: chronic inflammation isn't a life sentence. It's something we can control with the right diet and lifestyle choices. By incorporating more omega-3s into your daily routine – through foods like salmon, walnuts, chia seeds, and high-quality supplements – you're giving your body what it needs to keep inflammation in check and slow the aging process.

As Dr. Andrew Weil, a leader in integrative medicine, says, "The good news is that chronic inflammation can be controlled. And the best way to do that is through diet – specifically by increasing your intake of anti-inflammatory omega-3 fatty acids."

So, when you think about aging, don't just focus on the number of years – think about the quality of those years. Omega-3s, by reducing inflammation, help you age more gracefully, protect your cells, and keep your body functioning optimally for as long as possible.

Case Studies: Cultures with High Omega-3 Intake and Long Lifespans

When we talk about the impact of omega-3s on health and longevity, we don't have to rely on theory alone. Some of the most compelling evidence comes from real-world case studies of cultures that have naturally high omega-3 intake – and the long, healthy lives they live as a result. These cultures offer us a window into what's possible when we fuel our bodies with the right nutrients, and the results are nothing short of remarkable.

Let's take a look at a few key examples.

1. The Inuit of Greenland

One of the most well-known case studies comes from the Inuit population of Greenland. For centuries, the traditional Inuit diet has been rich in fatty fish, seals, and whales – all of which are incredibly high in omega-3s, particularly EPA and DHA. Despite a diet that's also high in fat, the Inuit have historically had some of the lowest rates of heart disease in the world.

How is this possible? Researchers have found that the high levels of omega-3s in their diet play a protective role, reducing inflammation, keeping blood pressure low, and preventing the buildup of harmful cholesterol in the arteries.

Dr. Jorn Dyerberg, a Danish scientist who was one of the first to study the Inuit diet said, "The high intake of omega-3 fatty acids from fish oils in the Inuit diet results in a blood lipid profile that protects against heart disease, despite their high fat consumption."

What's particularly fascinating about the Inuit is that they managed to maintain this low risk of heart disease without modern medicine, simply through their diet. While lifestyle factors like physical activity certainly play a role, the omega-3s they consumed consistently helped keep inflammation and cardiovascular risk factors in check. It's a powerful example of how the right fats can protect the heart and promote longevity.

2. The Japanese and the Okinawans

Japan, and in particular the island of Okinawa, is another culture that demonstrates the longevity benefits of omega-3s. Japan has one of the highest life expectancies in the world, and the Okinawans are famous for having an extraordinarily high number of centenarians – people who live to be 100 years old or more.

What's one of the major dietary factors that set the Japanese apart?

Their regular consumption of omega-3-rich fish like salmon, mackerel, and sardines. Omega-3s are a staple in the Japanese diet, and this high intake is linked to their low rates of heart disease, stroke, and certain cancers.

Researchers believe the omega-3s in their diet help protect against inflammation, maintain brain health, and support cardiovascular function. The connection between omega-3s and the long, healthy lives of the Okinawans is no coincidence.

Dr. Bradley Willcox, a gerontologist and co-author of 'The Okinawa Program' notes, "The Okinawan diet is low in calories but dense in nutrients, especially omega-3s from fish and other sources. This helps keep inflammation at bay and protects against age-related diseases, allowing them to live longer, healthier lives."

What's particularly inspiring about the Okinawans is that they not only live long lives, but they also enjoy good health well into old age. Their omega-3-rich diet helps protect their hearts and brains, reducing their risk of the chronic diseases that often come with aging.

3. The Mediterranean Diet

We can't talk about longevity without mentioning the Mediterranean diet, which is widely regarded as one of the healthiest in the world. Countries like Greece and Italy have lower rates of heart disease, obesity, and diabetes, and a big part of that is due to the traditional Mediterranean diet, which is rich in omega-3s from fish, nuts, seeds, and olive oil.

One of the key components of the Mediterranean diet is a high intake of fatty fish like sardines and anchovies, which are packed with omega-3s. Combined with other healthy fats from olive oil and a diet high in fruits, vegetables, and whole grains, this creates a nutrient profile that promotes heart health and reduces inflammation throughout the body.

Studies have shown that people who follow the Mediterranean diet not only have lower rates of chronic disease but also live longer, healthier lives. It's not just about longevity – it's about quality of life.

Dr. Walter Willett, a professor of epidemiology and nutrition at

Harvard said, "The Mediterranean diet, with its focus on omega-3-rich fish, healthy fats, and plant-based foods, is one of the best diets for promoting longevity and preventing chronic disease. It offers a model for how we can eat to live longer, healthier lives."

The Mediterranean diet, like the diets of the Inuit and the Japanese, emphasizes the power of omega-3s to protect our cells, reduce inflammation, and promote long-term health. It's a way of eating that's rooted in tradition but backed by modern science.

Metabolic Typing and Personalized Nutrition

While the Mediterranean diet has an impressive track record, particularly when it comes to heart health and healthy fats, it's important to recognize that not every diet works for every person. This is where the concept of metabolic typing comes into play.

Metabolic typing is a nutritional approach that suggests we all have different genetic and biochemical needs. It helps us understand if we're protein dominant, carb dominant, or a mixed type. A person with a protein-dominant metabolic type, for example, may thrive on a diet that includes more protein and healthy fats, while someone who is carb-dominant may feel their best on a diet with more plant-based foods and carbohydrates.

The Mediterranean diet, while rich in healthy fats, vegetables, and lean proteins, might not provide the same level of "horsepower" that a protein-dominant metabolic type requires for optimal health. However, when it comes to the conversation surrounding healthy fats – particularly the inclusion of omega-3s and monounsaturated fats from olive oil – the Mediterranean diet shines.

It's a reminder that nutrition is not one-size-fits-all. Understanding your metabolic type can help you tailor your diet to better suit your body's needs. But for those looking to optimize their intake of healthy fats, the Mediterranean diet is certainly a strong foundation to build from.

4. The Icarians of Greece

Another fascinating case study comes from the island of Ikaria, often referred to as "The Island Where People Forget to Die." The people of Ikaria have some of the highest longevity rates in the world, with an unusually high percentage of their population living well into their 90s and beyond.

Much like the Okinawans, the Icarians' diet is naturally rich in omega-3s, particularly from wild greens, nuts, and oily fish. Their traditional diet also includes high-quality olive oil, another source of healthy fats. This combination helps keep inflammation low, which is one of the keys to their long lives.

What's inspiring about the Icarians is that they don't just live longer – they live better. Chronic diseases like heart disease, cancer, and dementia are much less common, and they remain active and engaged in their community well into old age.

Dan Buettner, author of 'The Blue Zones', which examines the world's longest-living cultures said, "The Icarians' diet is rich in anti-inflammatory foods, particularly omega-3s, which helps them stay healthy and active long into their later years."

The Takeaway: What We Can Learn from These Cultures

When we look at these cultures – the Inuit, the Japanese, the Mediterraneans, and the Icarians – a common thread emerges. They all have diets that are naturally high in omega-3s, and this has a profound impact on their health and longevity. Whether it's protecting their hearts, reducing inflammation, or supporting cognitive function, omega-3s are a key factor in helping them live long, healthy lives.

And the beauty of it is that these diets aren't about deprivation. They're about abundance – enjoying nutrient-dense foods that nourish the body and promote well-being. For Sarah, and for so many others who feel stuck in the fast-food cycle, this is a hopeful message. It's not about making drastic changes overnight – it's about adding more of the good stuff, more omega-3s, and watching the benefits unfold over time.

As we learn from these cultures, we see that longevity isn't just about genetics or luck. It's about the choices we make every day – the food we eat, the way we care for our bodies, and how we nourish ourselves. Omega-3s are a crucial part of that equation, and by incorporating them into our lives, we can give ourselves the best possible chance for a long, healthy future.

Practical Steps: Balancing Omega-3s for a Longer, Healthier Life

As we wrap up this chapter on omega-3s and longevity, it's important to remember that while the science behind omega-3s is fascinating, it's the practical steps we take that make the real difference in our lives. Fortunately, balancing your omega-3 intake doesn't have to be complicated. Small, intentional changes can have a profound impact on your health and longevity.

The first thing I tell my patients, like Sarah, is to start by looking at their current diet. Often, the biggest issue isn't just a lack of omega-3s – it's the overwhelming presence of omega-6 fats from processed foods, seed oils, and takeout meals. By making a few simple swaps, you can begin to shift that balance back in your favor.

1. Eat More Omega-3-Rich Foods

The easiest and most natural way to increase your omega-3 intake is to eat more omega-3-rich foods. This includes fatty fish like salmon, mackerel, sardines, and herring, as well as plant-based sources like chia seeds, flaxseeds, and walnuts. Adding these foods to your diet on a regular basis ensures your body gets the essential fats it needs to thrive.

Dr. Frank Hu, professor of nutrition and epidemiology at Harvard points out, "One of the best ways to protect your heart and promote overall health is by increasing your intake of omega-3-rich foods. These fats reduce inflammation, improve blood flow, and promote longevity."

Make it a goal to incorporate fatty fish into your meals at least twice a week. If you're vegetarian or prefer plant-based options, focus on chia seeds, flaxseeds, and algae-based supplements, which are excellent sources of omega-3s.

2. Reduce Omega-6 Intake

Balancing your omega-3s also means reducing your intake of omega-6s. Remember, omega-6 fatty acids aren't inherently bad, but when consumed in excess – as they often are in the Standard American Diet – they can contribute to chronic inflammation. Processed foods, fried foods, and snacks made with seed oils like soybean, corn, and sunflower oil are the biggest culprits.

A simple way to make a big difference is to avoid processed and fried foods and cook with healthier oils like olive oil or avocado oil, which are rich in monounsaturated fats and won't throw off your omega balance.

Dr. David Katz, a leading voice in preventive medicine reminds us, "The goal isn't to eliminate omega-6s altogether but to create a better balance by reducing their dominance in our diets and increasing our intake of omega-3s."

3. Consider Omega-3 Supplements

If getting enough omega-3s through diet alone feels like a challenge, especially in today's fast-paced world, supplements can help fill the gap. Fish oil supplements are one of the most common and effective ways to boost your omega-3 intake. If you prefer a plant-based option, look for algae-based omega-3 supplements, which provide DHA and EPA without the need for fish.

Just be sure to choose a high-quality supplement. Look for brands that are third-party tested for purity and potency, ensuring you're getting the beneficial omega-3s without contaminants like mercury.

Dr. Joseph Maroon, a neurosurgeon and author of 'The Longevity Factor' emphasizes, "Omega-3 supplements can play a key role in promoting long-term health and reducing inflammation, especially when it's difficult to get enough from your diet alone."

4. Mind Your Ratios

While increasing your intake of omega-3s is essential, paying attention to the overall balance of omega-3 to omega-6 is equally important. One of the best ways to do this is by tracking what you eat. Apps and online tools can help you monitor your omega-3 and omega-6 intake, giving you a clearer picture of where adjustments are needed.

You don't have to aim for a perfect 1:1 ratio right away, but every small step toward reducing omega-6s and increasing omega-3s will benefit your health.

5. Be Consistent

The key to long-term health is consistency. It's not about doing everything perfectly all the time; it's about making incremental changes that you can stick with. The more you incorporate omega-3-rich foods into your diet, the more your body will thank you. Over time, you'll start to notice the benefits – better energy, reduced inflammation, and a stronger sense of well-being.

Dr. Andrew Stoll, a psychiatrist and expert in the use of omega-3s in brain health puts it simply, "Omega-3s are not a quick fix, but a long-term investment in your health. The more consistently you make them a part of your life, the greater the benefits."

A Hopeful Outlook

For Sarah, these practical steps felt doable – small changes that could make a big difference in her health and the health of her family. By focusing on balance, not perfection, she began to see the positive impact of omega-3s on her energy, her mood, and even her joint pain.

And the best part? You don't have to overhaul your life to see these benefits either. Start with one meal, one supplement, or one choice at a time. As you continue to make these adjustments, you're not just adding years to your life – you're adding quality to those years.

Balancing your fats is one of the most important investments you can make in your health. It's not about deprivation or strict rules; it's about giving your body what it needs to function at its best at a cellular level, which we will talk about in the next chapter. By incorporating more omega-3s and reducing the overload of omega-6s, you'll be taking practical steps toward a longer, healthier life – one filled with vitality and the ability to live fully each and every day.

three
cellular health – the foundation of longevity

AS WE DELVE DEEPER into the science of longevity and wellness, it's essential to start at the most fundamental level—the cell. The health of our cells determines the health of our bodies in ways that are both immediate and profound, impacting everything from our energy levels to the aging of our skin. For Sarah, this became strikingly clear as she embarked on her journey to balance her intake of omega-3 and omega-6 fatty acids.

When Sarah first came to see me, she was frustrated with her skin—dry, flaky, and prematurely aging, which she felt was just another sign of her deteriorating health. She hoped for improvement but wasn't sure where to start. As she began to integrate more omega-3-rich foods into her diet, something remarkable happened. Not only did her energy levels and joint health improve, but so did the health of her skin. It regained elasticity and moisture, becoming more radiant and youthful. The change was not just cosmetic; her skin, the largest organ of her body, had become a visible reflection of her improving cellular health.

This transformation is a testament to the power of cellular nutrition —a concept that underpins our entire approach to health and longevity. By nourishing our cells with the right nutrients, we can literally transform our bodies from the inside out.

How Omega-3s Impact Cellular Membranes

At the heart of cellular health is the cell membrane. This vital structure acts as the gatekeeper for the cell, controlling what enters and exits and facilitating communication between cells. The integrity and functionality of cell membranes are crucial for overall health, and this is where omega-3 fatty acids play a pivotal role.

Omega-3 fatty acids, particularly EPA and DHA, are integral components of cell membranes throughout the body. They help maintain the fluidity and flexibility of cell membranes, which is essential for cell signaling, nutrient uptake, and waste removal. When cell membranes are healthy, cells can communicate effectively and operate efficiently, leading to better health at every level of the body.

Dr. Bruce Holub, a university professor emeritus of nutritional sciences, emphasizes the importance of these fatty acids, "Omega-3 fatty acids are not just additives to our diet; they are integral to cell membrane structure and function, profoundly influencing cell behavior and health."

These fatty acids also play a critical role in the formation of lipid rafts—small, specialized areas within the cell membrane that are crucial for cellular signaling pathways. By influencing these pathways, omega-3s can affect how cells respond to various signals, including those involved in inflammation, survival, and cell death.

The impact of omega-3s on cellular membranes also extends to their anti-inflammatory properties. By incorporating into cell membranes, omega-3 fatty acids help modulate the activity of enzymes involved in inflammation, such as cyclooxygenase (COX) and lipoxygenase (LOX). This modulation can reduce the production of inflammatory molecules, leading to decreased inflammation throughout the body.

Moreover, the fluidity of cell membranes enhanced by omega-3s is crucial for the proper functioning of proteins embedded in the membrane, including receptors, enzymes, and ion channels. This fluidity allows for better transmission of signals across the membrane and more efficient cellular responses, which is vital for maintaining homeostasis and preventing chronic diseases.

Dr. Michael Crawford, a leading researcher in brain biochemistry, points out the broader implications of these effects, "The brain is especially rich in omega-3 fatty acids, which are essential for cognitive function and brain health. The impact of omega-3s on cell membranes throughout the body helps explain their profound effects on overall health and longevity."

As we continue to explore the cellular foundations of health, it becomes clear that omega-3 fatty acids are not just beneficial but essential for maintaining the structure and function of our cells. For Sarah, seeing the benefits of omega-3s manifest in her skin was just the beginning. Her journey toward better health at the cellular level is a powerful reminder of how deeply our diet can influence our biological processes and, ultimately, our lifespan.

This exploration of cellular health is not just about understanding how our bodies work—it's about taking actionable steps to improve our health from the inside out. By ensuring our cells have the right types of fats, like omega-3s, we're not just supporting individual cell functions—we're promoting a body that can heal, regenerate, and thrive for years to come.

Omega-3 and Mitochondrial Health: Boosting Energy at the Cellular Level

Mitochondria, often described as the "powerhouses of the cell," are crucial for converting the energy we consume into a form that our cells can use. These organelles play a pivotal role not just in energy production but in overall cellular health and longevity. The health of our mitochondria directly impacts our energy levels, metabolic health, and the aging process itself. This is a concept that Dr. Casey Means discusses at length in her book 'Good Energy', where she emphasizes the critical importance of mitochondrial health for maintaining vitality and well-being.

For Sarah and her children, understanding the role of omega-3 fatty acids in supporting mitochondrial function has been a game-changer. After incorporating more omega-3-rich foods into their diet, they noticed an uptick in their energy levels and overall vitality—a tangible sign of improved mitochondrial function.

The Role of Omega-3s in Mitochondrial Function

Omega-3 fatty acids, particularly docosahexaenoic acid (DHA), play a direct role in the health and efficiency of mitochondria. DHA is a major structural component of the membranes that surround mitochondria. Its presence in these membranes helps maintain their integrity and fluidity, which is crucial for optimal mitochondrial function.

Dr. Casey Means points out: "Mitochondria are not just the energy producers in our cells; they are also key to controlling the fate of cells and therefore our overall health and longevity. Omega-3 fatty acids help ensure that mitochondrial membranes remain functional and efficient, directly influencing our energy levels and capacity for healthy aging."

By integrating into mitochondrial membranes, omega-3s ensure that these membranes remain permeable and fluid. This fluidity is essential for the transport of proteins and nutrients into and out of the mitochondria, processes that are vital for energy production.

Omega-3s and Energy Production

One of the key functions of mitochondria is to produce ATP (adenosine triphosphate), the energy currency of the cell. Omega-3 fatty acids have been shown to enhance the biochemical pathways that generate ATP. This not only boosts energy at the cellular level but also improves overall vitality and supports the body's energy demands throughout the day.

As Sarah and her children began to experience, increased dietary intake of omega-3s translated into more sustained energy levels, less fatigue, and an enhanced ability to engage in daily activities. This was particularly noticeable in the children, who reported feeling more alert and energetic at school.

Reducing Oxidative Stress

Mitochondria are also a major site of oxidative stress due to the high levels of reactive oxygen species (ROS) they produce. While ROS are normal byproducts of metabolism, excessive ROS can damage cells and contribute to aging and disease. Omega-3 fatty acids have been shown to exert antioxidant effects, helping to neutralize ROS and reduce oxidative stress within mitochondria.

Dr. Elizabeth Blackburn, a Nobel laureate whose research focuses on telomeres and aging suggests, "Antioxidants play a critical role in protecting mitochondrial function and extending the lifespan of cells. Omega-3s contribute to this protective effect, helping to mitigate the aging process at the cellular level."

For Sarah, this meant not only feeling more energetic but also seeing visible signs of health improvement, such as better skin health and reduced signs of aging—outcomes that are deeply connected to the health of her mitochondria.

The Broader Impact of Healthy Mitochondria

The benefits of omega-3 fatty acids extend far beyond mere energy production. By supporting mitochondrial health, omega-3s help enhance metabolic efficiency, reduce systemic inflammation, and play a key role in cellular repair and maintenance. For anyone looking to boost their energy and promote long-term health, focusing on mitochondrial health through adequate intake of omega-3s is a vital strategy.

As Dr. Casey Means aptly puts it, "Optimizing our diet for mitochondrial health, particularly through the consumption of omega-3s, isn't just about boosting energy—it's about setting a foundation for a longer, healthier life."

For Sarah and her family, the journey toward better health continues to be fueled by these essential nutrients, reflecting a broader commitment to living well and thriving through the power of informed nutritional choices.

Reducing Oxidative Stress: The Role of Fats in Cellular Protection

Oxidative stress is a pervasive issue, one that affects our cells every day as a result of normal metabolic processes, environmental pollutants, and lifestyle factors like diet and stress. It is characterized by an imbalance between the production of reactive oxygen species (ROS) and the body's ability to counteract or detoxify their harmful effects through antioxidants. The role of dietary fats, particularly omega-3 fatty acids, in managing and mitigating oxidative stress, is profound and deserves a focused exploration.

Understanding Oxidative Stress

At its core, oxidative stress is about imbalance. ROS are chemically reactive molecules containing oxygen. While they are normal byproducts of cellular metabolism and play roles in cell signaling and homeostasis, excessive ROS can lead to cell damage, contributing to aging and various diseases, including cancer, cardiovascular diseases, and neurodegenerative disorders.

Dr. Rhonda Patrick, a biomedical scientist known for her research on nutritional health, explains, "Oxidative stress occurs when there's an imbalance between free radical generation and the body's ability to fight them off. Too much oxidative stress can accelerate aging and damage DNA, proteins, and other cellular structures."

The Role of Omega-3 Fatty Acids

Omega-3 fatty acids, particularly eicosapentaenoic acid (EPA) and docosahexaenoic acid (DHA), are more than just building blocks for cell membranes—they also play a crucial role in reducing oxidative stress. These fatty acids can help enhance the body's own antioxidant defenses, primarily through their anti-inflammatory properties.

Omega-3s influence oxidative stress indirectly by modulating the production of inflammatory cytokines and enzymes that generate ROS. By reducing inflammation, less ROS is produced, which consequently lowers oxidative stress. Furthermore, omega-3 fatty acids can directly scavenge ROS, neutralizing these harmful molecules before they cause cellular damage.

Dr. Joseph Hibbeln from the National Institutes of Health points out, "The anti-inflammatory effects of omega-3 fatty acids help reduce the production of molecules and substances linked to inflammation and oxidative stress. This is key to protecting cellular health and preventing chronic diseases."

Dietary Strategies to Combat Oxidative Stress

For Sarah and her family, understanding the relationship between diet and oxidative stress has been eye-opening. By incorporating omega-3-rich foods into their diet, they've not only improved their overall health but have also taken a proactive step in combating oxidative stress. Here are some practical dietary strategies:

1. Increase Omega-3 Intake: Incorporating foods rich in omega-3s, like fatty fish, flaxseeds, chia seeds, and walnuts, can boost the body's natural antioxidant defenses. For those who find it challenging to get enough omega-3s from diet alone, high-quality supplements can be an effective alternative.

2. Balance Fat Intake: While increasing omega-3s, it's also important to reduce intake of omega-6 fats, which are prevalent in processed foods and can promote oxidative stress if consumed in excess.

3. Antioxidant-Rich Foods: Beyond fats, consuming a diet rich in other antioxidants like vitamins C and E, selenium, and flavonoids found in fruits and vegetables can further help in neutralizing ROS.

4. Spices and Herbs: Incorporating spices like turmeric, which contains curcumin, and herbs like ginger can also enhance the body's antioxidant capacity.

The Broader Implications of Reduced Oxidative Stress

Reducing oxidative stress is a cornerstone of the 100+Living Plan, underscoring the profound connection between our cellular health and overall vitality. By managing oxidative stress, we actively combat the cellular damage that can accelerate aging and contribute to chronic diseases.

As Sarah began to see improvements in her skin health and overall energy levels, the connection between dietary choices and cellular health became clear. For her children, adopting these dietary habits early on not only boosts their current health but also sets the foundation for a healthier future.

Dr. Walter Willett, professor at Harvard School of Public Health, reinforces this approach, "A diet that is rich in omega-3 fatty acids and antioxidants is not just good for your heart; it's a solid strategy for protecting your cells against oxidative stress, reducing the risk of chronic diseases, and maintaining good health as you age."

Managing oxidative stress through diet, particularly by adjusting the types and amounts of fats we consume, offers a powerful tool for protecting our cells and maintaining long-term health. For Sarah and many others, making informed choices about dietary fats is not just about preventing disease—it's about empowering a vibrant, active life, well into the future. This proactive approach to diet underscores the profound impact that nutrients like omega-3s have on our health at the most fundamental cellular level.

Supporting Your Cells: How to Optimize Fat Intake

Optimizing fat intake is essential for maintaining cellular health and ensuring the smooth functioning of our bodies. But it's not just about choosing the right types of fats—how and when we consume these fats can also significantly impact their benefits. This section explores practical strategies for optimizing fat intake to support cellular health, guided by the principles of the 100+Living Plan.

Choosing the Right Fats

The first step in supporting your cells through diet is ensuring you're consuming the right types of fats. Focus on incorporating a balance of healthy fats that include:

1. Omega-3 Fatty Acids: Found in fatty fish like salmon, mackerel, and sardines, as well as in flaxseeds, chia seeds, and walnuts. These fats are crucial for reducing inflammation and supporting cell membrane integrity.

2. Monounsaturated Fats: Found in olive oil, avocados, and nuts.

These fats help improve heart health and provide essential nutrients for cell function.

3. Saturated Fats: While they should be consumed in moderation, saturated fats from sources like coconut oil and grass-fed butter play a role in cellular health, contributing to the integrity of cell membranes.

Dr. Mark Hyman, a functional medicine expert, notes, "Fat is not just a fuel source. It's the building block of your cell membranes, the functioning of your brain and hormones. The key is to choose the right fats and integrate them wisely into your diet."

Optimizing Fat Consumption for Nutrient Absorption

The order in which we consume macronutrients—fats, proteins, and carbohydrates—can affect how well our bodies absorb and utilize these nutrients. To optimize nutrient absorption, particularly of fat-soluble vitamins (A, D, E, and K), include a healthy fat source at each meal. This not only ensures better absorption of vitamins but also helps stabilize blood sugar levels.

Consuming Fats with Meals

Integrating fats into your meals can help slow the absorption of carbohydrates, leading to a more gradual rise in blood sugar levels. For optimal health, start your meals with a serving of vegetables, followed by protein, and then add healthy fats. This sequence can enhance satiety and further support metabolic health.

Dr. Jason Fung, a leading expert in metabolism, suggests, "Consuming healthy fats after other macronutrients can help in slowing digestion and absorption, offering more sustained energy and preventing spikes in blood sugar, which is crucial for maintaining optimal metabolic function."

Practical Tips for Daily Fat Intake

1. Breakfast: Start your day with eggs cooked in olive oil or avocado oil, served with avocado slices or a small handful of nuts.

2. Lunch: Include a salad dressed with olive oil and vinegar, topped with seeds like pumpkin or sunflower for an additional omega-3 boost.

3. Dinner: Prepare fatty fish like salmon several times a week, accompanied by steamed vegetables drizzled with olive oil or a pat of grass-fed butter.

4. Snacks: Opt for raw nuts or yogurt mixed with chia seeds to keep your energy levels stable throughout the day.

By focusing on the quality, balance, and timing of fat consumption, we can maximize the health benefits of dietary fats. These strategies not only support cellular health but also contribute to overall wellness, energy levels, and longevity. As we incorporate these practices into our daily lives, we empower our bodies to function optimally, reinforcing the core principles of the 100+Living Plan.

Dr. Sarah Hallberg, an advocate for dietary wellness sums it up, "Remember, fat is a vital nutrient. Embracing good fats in your diet can transform your health, giving your cells the tools they need to thrive. It's about making informed choices that support not just longevity but also the quality of your life."

This integrative approach ensures that each cell in your body is nourished and protected, paving the way for a vibrant and healthy future.

four

brain and neurological health – the omega-3 connection

AS A PRACTITIONER SPECIALIZING in neurologically based healthcare, I've witnessed firsthand the profound impact that brain health has on the entire body. The health of your brain, spinal cord, and spinal nerves indeed dictates the function and well-being of every other cell, tissue, and organ in your body. This interconnectedness is fundamental to understanding how we approach healing and wellness, emphasizing that a well-functioning nervous system is crucial for overall health.

Sarah's journey to my clinic was marked by a series of frustrations with traditional medical approaches. She had seen multiple doctors and therapists, but her health issues persisted until we began to fully assess and address her neurological deficiencies. It wasn't just about alleviating symptoms; it was about restoring the underlying health of her nervous system, which we achieved by integrating specific nutritional strategies, particularly focusing on omega-3 fatty acids. This approach not only transformed Sarah's health but also illuminated the critical role that these fats play in neurological health.

In addition to enhancing Sarah's diet with critical omega-3 fatty acids to bolster her neurological health, we also tackled specific structural challenges contributing to tensile stress on her spinal cord and spinal nerves, as Sarah was diagnosed with Adult Spinal Deformity (ASD). Addressing these structural issues was crucial, as they directly impact the integrity and functionality of the neurological system, which in turn influences overall health and well-being. This comprehensive approach was a key component of Sarah's 100+Living Plan, aiming not just to alleviate symptoms but to restore and optimize health at every level.

For those interested in a deeper understanding of ASD and its implications on health, I delve into this topic extensively in my first book of the 100+ series. The book provides a detailed exploration of postural and structural deformities encompassed within the ASD umbrella, offering step-by-step insights into managing and improving these conditions. This holistic perspective is vital for anyone seeking to achieve a profound and lasting impact on their health, embodying the essence of the 100+Living Plan that has guided Sarah and many others toward reclaiming their vitality and longevity.

Back to Omega 3's

This chapter delves into the essential relationship between omega-3 fatty acids, particularly docosahexaenoic acid (DHA), and brain health. We'll explore how these vital nutrients support neurological function, contribute to brain development, and protect against cognitive decline, offering a beacon of hope for maintaining brain health throughout life.

DHA: The Brain's Essential Fat

Docosahexaenoic acid (DHA) is more than just another nutrient; it is fundamental to the structure and function of the human brain. Representing about 97% of the omega-3 fats in the brain and 25% of its total fat content, DHA is critical for optimal brain health and function.

Structural Role of DHA

DHA is a primary building block of the cerebral cortex, the part of the brain responsible for memory, emotion, attention, and creativity. It's also crucial for the development of the eye's retina. Its structural role is not merely passive; DHA makes up part of the cell membranes and contributes to the fluidity and function of these membranes, which is essential for the transmission of brain signals.

Dr. Michael Crawford, a leading figure in brain chemistry and nutrition, asserts, "The brain is fat's most greedy organ. DHA provides the fluidity required for fast nerve transmission. Without it, you can have all the right signals, all the right ideas, but they won't be transmitted effectively inside the brain."

Cognitive Health and Aging

The implications of DHA for cognitive health are far-reaching, especially as we age. Numerous studies have linked higher DHA levels with a reduced risk of cognitive decline and dementia. This protective effect is thought to arise from DHA's ability to reduce oxidative stress, inflammation, and the formation of beta-amyloid plaques, which are hallmarks of Alzheimer's disease.

Mental Health Benefits

Beyond aging, DHA is also critically involved in mental health. Research suggests that adequate levels of DHA can improve mood disorders, such as depression and anxiety. Its anti-inflammatory effects are particularly beneficial, considering the growing evidence linking inflammation to mental health issues.

Dr. Joseph Hibbeln from the National Institutes of Health highlights this point, "Clinical trials have shown that DHA supplementation decreases depression symptoms significantly. It's not just good for the body but crucial for the brain and mental health."

Supporting Neurological Health with DHA

Ensuring adequate intake of DHA can be particularly beneficial for individuals like Sarah, whose neurological health needs support. This can be achieved through dietary sources such as fatty fish—salmon, mackerel, and sardines are excellent choices—and through high-quality fish oil supplements, ensuring that both the quantity and quality of DHA are sufficient to meet the body's needs.

For Sarah, integrating a diet high in DHA was a turning point in her treatment plan. It supported not just her neurological function but also her overall vitality, illustrating how central good fat intake is to comprehensive health strategies.

As we explore deeper into the neurological benefits of DHA, it becomes clear that this essential fat is a cornerstone of brain health. Whether you're looking to enhance cognitive function, protect against age-related decline, or improve mental well-being, DHA offers a pathway to achieving these goals. Its profound impact on brain structure and function exemplifies the powerful role nutrition plays in our neurological health, empowering us with strategies to support our brain throughout our lives.

Cognitive Decline and Dementia: How Omega-3s Slow Brain Aging

One of the most compelling areas of research in the realm of omega-3 fatty acids is their impact on the brain, particularly in the prevention and slowing of cognitive decline and dementia. As we age, our brains are susceptible to various forms of degeneration, but omega-3 fatty acids, especially docosahexaenoic acid (DHA), have shown promising potential in mitigating these effects.

Omega-3s and Brain Protection

DHA is not just a structural component of the brain; it plays a critical role in maintaining brain health and function. It influences brain processes by enhancing membrane fluidity, which is crucial for the proper functioning of neurotransmitter systems and signal transmission. This fluidity allows neurons to communicate effectively, a key factor in maintaining cognitive function as we age.

Dr. Gregory Cole, a neuroscientist specializing in Alzheimer's research, notes, "Omega-3 fatty acids, particularly DHA, are thought to help prevent Alzheimer's by reducing beta-amyloid plaques, known to be a hallmark of the disease. These fatty acids interfere with the processes that produce these harmful plaques, offering a protective shield for the brain cells."

Research on Omega-3s and Cognitive Health

Numerous studies have linked higher dietary intake of omega-3s with reduced rates of cognitive decline. Research indicates that individuals who regularly consume omega-3-rich foods or supplements have a slower rate of cognitive deterioration, often associated with aging and neurodegenerative diseases like Alzheimer's and Parkinson's.

A groundbreaking study published in the journal 'Neurology' found that higher levels of omega-3 fatty acids in the blood were associated with better brain structure and cognitive function in older adults. This correlation highlights the potential of omega-3s to not only maintain brain health but also improve it, even in later stages of life.

Mechanisms of Action

The mechanisms by which omega-3 fatty acids impact brain aging are multifaceted:

1. Anti-inflammatory effects: Omega-3s reduce the level of inflammation in the brain, which is linked to neurodegenerative diseases.

2. Antioxidant properties: These fatty acids help combat oxidative stress that damages brain cells.

3. Enhancing neuroplasticity: Omega-3s promote the growth of new neural connections, crucial for learning and memory.

Dr. Martha Clare Morris, a nutritional epidemiologist, explains, "The anti-inflammatory and antioxidant effects of omega-3 fatty acids are particularly important in the brain, where inflammation and oxidative stress are associated with cognitive decline. By modulating these processes, omega-3s help preserve cognitive functions and slow down brain aging."

Practical Application for Daily Life

Incorporating omega-3s into the diet can be a straightforward, practical step towards maintaining brain health:

1. Diet: Include fish like salmon, mackerel, and sardines in your diet multiple times per week.

2. Supplements: Consider high-quality omega-3 supplements if dietary sources are insufficient or unavailable. Personally, my supplements are the key to ensuing I get the ratio right in my life, not because I'm ordering take out but because I struggle with getting my meals in with my full schedule.

3. Whole-food approach: Combine omega-3 intake with other brain-healthy nutrients such as antioxidants from berries, nuts, and green leafy vegetables to maximize benefits.

For Sarah, integrating omega-3s into her daily routine was part of a broader strategy to enhance her neurological health, reflecting her commitment to the principles of the 100+Living Plan. By focusing on omega-3s, we not only aim to prolong life but also to enhance the quality of those extra years, ensuring that our brains remain as active and vibrant as possible.

As we continue to uncover more about the role of omega-3s in brain health, the hope is that more individuals will embrace these nutrients as a fundamental part of their diet, paving the way for healthier, more fulfilling golden years.

The Neurological Benefits: Mood, Memory, and Mental Clarity of Getting Your Fats Right

In the realm of neurology, the profound impact of dietary fats, particularly omega-3 fatty acids, on brain function is increasingly evident. From enhancing cognitive recovery post-concussion to boosting mental clarity in aging populations, the right balance of fats is proving to be a cornerstone of neurological health. This section delves into how omega-3s, especially EPA (eicosapentaenoic acid) and DHA (docosahexaenoic acid), influence mood, memory, and mental clarity, supported by clinical evidence and expert insights.

Omega-3s and Cognitive Recovery

The role of omega-3s in cognitive recovery, particularly following traumatic brain injuries such as concussions, is garnering attention. DHA, a major component of brain tissue, has been shown to play a crucial role in repairing and regenerating neural cells.

Dr. Michael Lewis, an expert in brain health and recovery, emphasizes the importance of omega-3s post-injury, "When we look at brain health and recovery, omega-3 fatty acids can significantly influence the healing process. DHA helps rebuild damaged neural pathways, enhancing the recovery speed and extent following brain injuries." His research has demonstrated that high doses of omega-3 fatty acids can improve outcomes in patients suffering from acute and chronic brain injuries by reducing inflammation and promoting brain repair.

Enhancing Memory and Cognitive Function

Omega-3 fatty acids are also vital for memory enhancement and the preservation of cognitive function, particularly in older adults. Numerous studies have linked higher omega-3 intake with reductions in the rate of cognitive decline.

Dr. Elizabeth Coulson, a neuroscientist specializing in age-related cognitive deterioration, notes, "Omega-3 fatty acids are not just nutrients; they are essential components of brain health that directly contribute to memory preservation and cognitive agility in aging populations. Regular intake of these fats is associated with lower risks of developing Alzheimer's disease and other forms of dementia."

A pivotal study in the 'Journal of Alzheimer's Disease' reported that individuals with higher levels of omega-3 fatty acids in their diet had better cognitive performance and showed slower cognitive decline compared to those with lower levels.

Omega-3s for Mood Regulation

The impact of omega-3s extends beyond cognitive functions to include significant benefits for mental health, particularly in the modulation of mood disorders. The anti-inflammatory properties of EPA are believed to play a critical role in mood regulation by influencing neurotransmitter pathways and reducing neuroinflammation, which is often elevated in mood disorders such as depression and anxiety.

Dr. Uma Naidoo, a nutritional psychiatrist, states, "Integrating omega-3 fatty acids into the diet of patients dealing with depression has shown promising results, often comparable to the effects seen with conventional antidepressant treatments. EPA, in particular, has potent anti-inflammatory effects that help combat the inflammation seen in depressive states."

Clinical trials have supported the use of omega-3 supplements as adjunct therapy for depression, highlighting significant improvements in mood among participants who received high doses of EPA and DHA.

The neurological benefits of getting your fats right, particularly through the inclusion of omega-3 fatty acids, are profound. From enhancing cognitive recovery and supporting mental clarity to improving mood and overall mental health, omega-3s offer a foundational strategy for maintaining and enhancing neurological health. As evidenced in my clinical practice and supported by a growing body of research, these fats are not just building blocks of brain tissue; they are active players in promoting resilience and longevity in brain function.

Omega-3 Deficiency and Its Impact on Mental Health

In recent years, the connection between nutrition and mental health has become increasingly clear, with omega-3 fatty acids taking center stage in this discussion. Omega-3s, particularly EPA and DHA, are essential not only for physical health but also for maintaining mental well-being. When these essential fats are lacking in the diet, the consequences can be profound, leading to an increased risk of depression, anxiety, and even more severe mental health issues such as suicidal behavior.

The Link Between Omega-3 Deficiency and Mental Health Disorders

Omega-3 fatty acids play an integral role in the brain's structure and function. DHA, in particular, is a major structural component of neuronal membranes, helping to maintain membrane fluidity and facilitate communication between neurons. EPA, on the other hand, has been found to have potent anti-inflammatory effects, reducing neuroinflammation, which is increasingly linked to mental health disorders such as depression.

When omega-3 intake is insufficient, this can lead to an imbalance in brain chemistry and function. Low levels of omega-3s have been associated with reduced neurotransmitter activity, particularly of serotonin, the "feel-good" hormone that regulates mood. The result is often an increased susceptibility to depression and anxiety.

Dr. Andrew Stoll, a psychiatrist and researcher at Harvard Medical School, conducted groundbreaking research showing that omega-3 supplementation could significantly improve symptoms of depression, particularly in individuals with treatment-resistant depression. He states: "Omega-3 fatty acids can modulate serotonin levels, help stabilize mood, and reduce the severity of depressive episodes."

Global Data: Omega-6 to Omega-3 Ratios and Mental Health

One of the most telling pieces of evidence linking omega-3 deficiency to mental health comes from studies comparing dietary patterns across different countries. Research has shown that countries with diets high in omega-6 fatty acids—predominantly from processed vegetable oils—tend to have higher rates of mental health disorders, including depression, anxiety, and suicide.

A study published in the 'American Journal of Psychiatry' found that populations with higher omega-3 consumption, such as those in Japan and Iceland, have lower rates of depression and suicide compared to countries like the United States, where the ratio of omega-6 to omega-3 is heavily skewed in favor of omega-6 fats. This imbalance is largely due to the widespread use of processed oils and a lack of omega-3-rich foods in the typical Western diet.

Dr. Joseph Hibbeln, a neuroscientist at the National Institutes of Health and a leading researcher on the relationship between omega-3s and mental health, conducted an influential study on this topic. He notes, "There is a clear association between the ratio of omega-6 to omega-3 in the diet and the prevalence of major depression and suicide rates. Populations that consume more omega-6 fats, particularly from processed foods, have significantly higher rates of mental health disorders."

Omega-3 Deficiency and Suicide Risk

Perhaps the most alarming consequence of omega-3 deficiency is its association with suicide. A study published in 'The Journal of Clinical Psychiatry' found that individuals with lower levels of omega-3 fatty acids, particularly EPA, were more likely to experience suicidal thoughts and behaviors. The study pointed to the role of omega-3s in reducing inflammation and regulating mood, both of which are critical in preventing the mental health crises that often precede suicide.

Dr. Hibbeln's research into omega-3s and mental health also found that countries with lower levels of omega-3 consumption had significantly higher suicide rates. For example, countries like Japan, where fish (a rich source of omega-3s) is a dietary staple, have some of the lowest suicide rates globally, whereas countries with lower fish consumption and higher intake of processed omega-6-rich foods show a troubling rise in suicide rates.

How Omega-3s Protect Mental Health

Omega-3s protect mental health in several key ways:

Reducing Inflammation: Chronic inflammation in the brain is increasingly recognized as a contributor to mental health disorders. Omega-3s, particularly EPA, help reduce neuroinflammation, which is often elevated in individuals with depression and anxiety.

Balancing Neurotransmitters: Omega-3s modulate the function of neurotransmitters like serotonin and dopamine, both of which play a critical role in mood regulation, pleasure, and motivation. A deficiency in omega-3s can lead to dysregulation of these neurotransmitters, increasing the risk of mood disorders.

Promoting Neuroplasticity: DHA is crucial for neuroplasticity, the brain's ability to form new neural connections. This is particularly important in individuals recovering from trauma or mental health challenges, as neuroplasticity allows the brain to adapt, heal, and develop resilience.

Dr. Michael Crawford, a leading authority on brain chemistry, underscores the importance of omega-3s for mental health, "The brain's need for omega-3s cannot be overstated. They are essential for cognitive function, emotional regulation, and overall brain health. A deficiency creates a perfect storm for mental health issues to develop and persist."

Hope Through Dietary Change

While the consequences of omega-3 deficiency are serious, the hopeful message is that dietary change can significantly impact mental health. By rebalancing the intake of omega-6 and omega-3 fatty acids, individuals can support their mental well-being, reduce symptoms of depression and anxiety, and even prevent more severe mental health issues like suicidal thoughts.

For Sarah, addressing her omega-3 deficiency was one of the most important steps in her recovery. After struggling with anxiety and mood swings for years, she found that incorporating more omega-3-rich foods into her diet, such as fatty fish, flaxseeds, and walnuts, helped stabilize her mood and improve her overall mental clarity. The real key for consistency with Sarah was the addition of a high-quality fish oil supplement. Her greatest challenge was her work and home responsibilities. Those responsibilities didn't change when she walked through the door of my clinic, so for her to ensure her health continued to keep up with her full life, supplementation was the final piece of the plan.

I believe that Omega-3 deficiency is a silent yet significant contributor to the growing mental health crisis worldwide. From mood disorders to the risk of suicide, the lack of these essential fats in modern diets

has far-reaching implications. However, the solution is within reach. By making intentional changes to balance omega-6 and omega-3 intake, individuals can experience profound improvements in their mental health, mood stability, and overall emotional well-being. The science is clear: getting your fats right isn't just about physical health—it's a vital part of protecting and nurturing your mind.

a request for your honest feedback

Now that you are part way through my book I'd like to invite you to share your thoughts and experiences by leaving an honest review on Amazon. Your feedback is not only important to me but also instrumental in enhancing the overall quality of this book. I am committed to delivering content that goes above and beyond your expectations, and your insights play a crucial role in achieving this.

Reviews not only help prospective readers make informed decisions but also provide me with an opportunity to address any areas that may need further clarification or expansion. Your observations and suggestions are immensely valuable as I strive to create a resource that truly empowers and supports you on your health journey.

Your reviews enable me to refine the content, fill any gaps that may exist, and ensure that the information presented is accessible and applicable to a wide audience.

My commitment to you is to deliver more value than you expect from this book. Your feedback will not only help shape the future editions but also contribute to the creation of a community dedicated to positive change and holistic well-being.

Thank you again for investing your time with my book, I look forward to hearing your thoughts and insights. Together, we can make a difference in the lives of many.

Wishing you health and happiness,

Dr. J

five

cardiovascular health – the heart loves omega-3s

HEART HEALTH HAS ALWAYS BEEN personal for me. In my family, the men have been plagued by catastrophic heart issues—heart attacks, strokes, and sudden cardiac events that have taken loved ones too soon. I've watched as these conditions have not only shortened lives but also dramatically reduced quality of life. It's an all-too-common story, and I've made it my mission to ensure that it doesn't become my story.

I have no interest in dropping dead of a heart attack or living with heart disease that limits my ability to enjoy life. That's why I've taken a proactive approach to heart health, focusing heavily on preventing the same fate. Central to this prevention strategy is balancing my intake of omega-3 and omega-6 fats, which I've come to understand plays a critical role in protecting the cardiovascular system. This chapter is dedicated to sharing the science behind how omega-3s support heart health —and why making this balance a priority in your life can make all the difference.

The Cardiovascular System: How Omega-3s Support Heart Function

The heart is an incredible organ, pumping blood and delivering oxygen to every cell in our bodies. But like any other system in the body, it's heavily influenced by the nutrients we provide it. Omega-3 fatty acids, particularly EPA and DHA, are critical to heart health, helping to keep the cardiovascular system running smoothly and protecting against the very conditions that lead to heart attacks, strokes, and other life-threatening events.

One of the most important ways omega-3s support heart function is by balancing inflammation in the body. Chronic inflammation is a major driver of cardiovascular disease, and it's closely tied to an imbalance between omega-6 and omega-3 fatty acids. Omega-6s, which are abundant in processed foods and seed oils, promote inflammation when consumed in excess. In contrast, omega-3s are potent anti-inflammatory agents that help reduce the risk of heart disease by counteracting this inflammation.

Dr. Dariush Mozaffarian, a renowned cardiologist and nutrition scientist emphasizes, "Inflammation plays a key role in the development of cardiovascular disease, and omega-3s help reduce that inflammation, improving heart health and lowering the risk of heart attacks and strokes."

By balancing the omega-6 to omega-3 ratio, we can reduce inflammation in the arteries, lowering the likelihood of plaque buildup, which is the primary cause of heart attacks and strokes. This balance is essential because it directly affects how our blood vessels function. When inflammation is high, arteries stiffen, blood pressure rises, and the risk of clot formation increases—all of which contribute to cardiovascular events.

Improving Heart Rhythm and Reducing Arrhythmias

Another key benefit of omega-3s is their ability to improve heart rhythm. Heart arrhythmias—abnormal heart rhythms—are a significant risk factor for sudden cardiac death. Studies have shown that higher levels of omega-3s, particularly EPA and DHA, can help stabilize the heart's electrical activity, reducing the risk of arrhythmias.

Research published in the 'Circulation' journal has found that omega-3 supplementation can lower the risk of sudden cardiac death by improving heart rhythm stability. This is particularly important for people with a history of heart disease or those at risk of arrhythmias.

Dr. William Harris, an expert in omega-3s and cardiovascular health notes, "Omega-3 fatty acids help make the heart more resilient by improving the stability of the heart's electrical system. This reduces the risk of arrhythmias, which can lead to sudden cardiac death."

Lowering Blood Pressure and Triglycerides

Omega-3s also play a significant role in reducing two other major risk factors for heart disease: high blood pressure and elevated triglycerides. Studies have consistently shown that omega-3s can help lower blood pressure by improving the elasticity of blood vessels, allowing blood to flow more easily through the circulatory system.

In addition, omega-3s are well-known for their ability to lower triglyceride levels. High levels of triglycerides—fats found in the blood —are associated with an increased risk of heart disease. By reducing triglycerides, omega-3s help protect the heart and lower the risk of atherosclerosis, a condition in which plaque builds up in the arteries, leading to heart attacks and strokes.

The American Heart Association has endorsed omega-3 supplementation for individuals with high triglycerides, stating that "omega-3 fatty acids have been shown to significantly reduce triglyceride levels, a critical factor in lowering the risk of heart disease."

The Omega-3 and Omega-6 Balance for Heart Health

One of the most critical aspects of omega-3's protective effects on the heart is its ability to restore balance in the modern diet, which is typically overloaded with omega-6 fatty acids. While omega-6s aren't inherently bad, consuming too many without adequate omega-3s creates an inflammatory environment that increases the risk of heart disease.

Achieving the right balance between omega-3 and omega-6 is essential for protecting the cardiovascular system. A ratio skewed too heavily toward omega-6s can fuel inflammation, while increasing omega-3s helps shift the body back toward an anti-inflammatory state, promoting heart health and longevity.

Dr. Artemis Simopoulos, a leading expert on essential fatty acids states, "The optimal omega-6 to omega-3 ratio for heart health is around 2:1 or even 1:1. Unfortunately, the typical Western diet is more like 15:1 or 20:1, which is fueling the heart disease epidemic we see today."

By focusing on incorporating more omega-3-rich foods—such as fatty fish, flaxseeds, chia seeds, and walnuts—into your diet, while reducing omega-6-laden processed foods, you can create an environment where your heart can thrive.

A Hopeful Path Forward

For me, the decision to prioritize omega-3 intake isn't just about statistics or research papers—it's about ensuring that I live a long, healthy life, free from the heart issues that have affected the men in my family. I'm committed to doing everything I can to avoid the fate that has plagued them, and omega-3s are a crucial part of that strategy.

The science is clear: omega-3s offer powerful protection for the heart by reducing inflammation, stabilizing heart rhythms, lowering blood pressure, and improving the overall function of the cardiovascular system. By making small, intentional changes to your diet, you too can protect your heart and enjoy a longer, healthier life.

Omega-3s and Blood Pressure: Reducing the Risk of Hypertension

High blood pressure, or hypertension, is often referred to as the "silent killer" because it can quietly damage the heart, arteries, and other vital organs without obvious symptoms. It's one of the leading risk factors for heart disease and stroke, and managing it effectively is key to long-term cardiovascular health. Fortunately, omega-3 fatty acids, particularly EPA and DHA, have been shown to play a significant role in reducing blood pressure and improving overall heart function.

How Omega-3s Lower Blood Pressure

The connection between omega-3s and blood pressure lies in the ability of these fatty acids to improve the elasticity and flexibility of blood vessels. Omega-3s help dilate blood vessels, making it easier for blood to flow through them, which in turn reduces the pressure exerted on artery walls. This process is crucial for maintaining healthy blood pressure levels and preventing damage to the cardiovascular system.

Dr. Penny Kris-Etherton, a distinguished professor of nutrition at Penn State University, has conducted extensive research on omega-3s and heart health. She explains, "Omega-3s improve the function of the endothelium, the lining of blood vessels, helping them to relax and dilate more easily. This improves blood flow and lowers blood pressure, which is a critical factor in reducing the risk of heart attacks and strokes."

In addition to improving blood vessel function, omega-3s help reduce inflammation and decrease the production of substances that can cause blood vessels to constrict, such as thromboxane and endothelin. By lowering levels of these substances, omega-3s help keep blood pressure in check and reduce the strain on the heart.

The Evidence on Omega-3s and Hypertension

Several studies have demonstrated the blood pressure-lowering effects of omega-3 fatty acids. A meta-analysis published in the 'American Journal of Hypertension' reviewed 70 randomized controlled trials and found that individuals who consumed omega-3 supplements or increased their intake of fatty fish experienced significant reductions in both systolic and diastolic blood pressure.

The benefits were particularly noticeable in individuals with high blood pressure, as well as those who were overweight or older—populations most at risk for hypertension. According to the study, people with hypertension saw an average reduction of 4.5 mm Hg in systolic blood pressure and 3 mm Hg in diastolic blood pressure when they increased their omega-3 intake.

Dr. Harris, a leading expert on omega-3s, explains the importance of these findings: "Even modest reductions in blood pressure can lead to meaningful reductions in cardiovascular risk. For individuals with hypertension, omega-3s offer a natural way to support heart health and reduce the need for more aggressive medical interventions."

A Natural Approach to Managing Blood Pressure

One of the most hopeful aspects of omega-3s' effect on blood pressure is that they offer a natural, non-pharmaceutical approach to managing hypertension. While medications can certainly play a role, incorporating omega-3-rich foods or supplements into the diet is an accessible and sustainable strategy for long-term heart health.

In fact, the American Heart Association recommends eating at least two servings of fatty fish per week to support heart health and lower blood pressure. Foods such as salmon, mackerel, sardines, and flaxseeds are excellent sources of omega-3s and can easily be incorporated into daily meals.

Practical Steps for Lowering Blood Pressure with Omega-3s

For individuals like Sarah, who came to me with concerns about her blood pressure and overall heart health, increasing her omega-3 intake was a simple yet powerful step toward managing her hypertension. Here are a few practical ways to get started and as you will see the recommendations in each chapter have some common elements, it really is simpler than you think, so here's my short list:

1. Eat More Fatty Fish: Aim for at least two servings of fatty fish per week, such as salmon, mackerel, sardines, or herring. These are among the richest sources of EPA and DHA.

2. Consider Omega-3 Supplements: If it's difficult to consume enough omega-3s through diet alone, high-quality fish oil supplements can be a convenient and effective option.

3. Add Flaxseeds or Chia Seeds: For plant-based omega-3s, add ground flaxseeds or chia seeds to smoothies, salads, or oatmeal. These are good sources of ALA (alpha-linolenic acid), which the body can convert into EPA and DHA.

4. Reduce Omega-6s: Lowering your intake of processed foods and vegetable oils that are high in omega-6s can also help improve the omega-3 to omega-6 ratio, supporting healthy blood pressure levels.

Omega-3s offer an incredible advantage for heart health, and their ability to naturally reduce blood pressure is just one of the many ways they protect the cardiovascular system. Whether you're managing existing hypertension or looking to prevent it, incorporating more omega-3s into your diet is a straightforward, effective strategy.

As research continues to reveal the wide-ranging benefits of these essential fatty acids, the message remains clear: by getting your fats right, you can support your heart, lower your blood pressure, and take meaningful steps toward a longer, healthier life.

Heart Disease Prevention: The Omega-3 to Omega-6 Balance

When it comes to heart disease prevention, we often hear about reducing saturated fat, watching cholesterol, or avoiding sodium. But one of the most important—and often overlooked—factors is the balance between omega-3 and omega-6 fatty acids in your diet. Think of this balance as the heart's secret weapon, one that can dramatically reduce inflammation, lower risk factors, and fortify your cardiovascular health. Yet, in the modern world, maintaining this balance requires intentional choices, especially in a landscape flooded with processed foods.

Many of us are unknowingly consuming too much omega-6 and not enough omega-3, creating an environment ripe for inflammation, which is a significant driver of heart disease. Omega-6 fats, found in many vegetable oils, processed snacks, and fast food, aren't inherently bad—our bodies need them in moderation. However, it's the overconsumption of omega-6s combined with a lack of omega-3s that shifts the body into a pro-inflammatory state. Omega-3s are the counterbalance. They are the anti-inflammatory warriors that help repair damaged blood vessels, stabilize heart rhythms, and reduce the risk of clotting.

Dr. William Harris, a well-known expert on omega-3 fatty acids, explains this balance perfectly, "It's not that omega-6 fats are 'bad' fats and omega-3s are 'good' fats, but it's the balance between the two that's key. Too much omega-6 and not enough omega-3 can tip the scales towards inflammation and heart disease."

Reframing the Omega Balance: A Lifestyle Shift, Not a Restriction

For many, the idea of maintaining the right omega-3 to omega-6 balance may seem like another dietary hurdle. But let's rethink it. Instead of viewing this as yet another restriction or "can't have," see it as an opportunity to elevate the quality of your diet—and by extension, your life.

You don't need to overhaul everything overnight or go to extreme measures to achieve this balance. Small, consistent adjustments will make a meaningful difference. It's about adding more of the foods that support your heart—salmon, mackerel, chia seeds, walnuts—and dialing back on the processed oils found in fast food, snack foods, and margarine. A good way to start is simply being more mindful of the oils you're using to cook or dress your salads. Choose olive oil over sunflower or soybean oil. Start incorporating omega-3-rich foods as staples rather than occasional treats.

Balancing Omega Fats Isn't Difficult—It's Empowering

Maintaining a better omega-3 to omega-6 ratio doesn't have to be complicated. It's not about following a rigid diet; it's about learning to make choices that nourish your body from the inside out. And once you start, the results can be incredibly empowering. You'll begin to feel better, notice more energy, and may even see improvements in cholesterol levels and blood pressure. You're giving your heart the tools it needs to thrive and resist the very conditions that might otherwise lead to heart disease.

One study published in the 'Journal of Nutrition' found that people with a better balance of omega-3 to omega-6 had a significant reduction in the risk of cardiovascular disease. The study highlighted the critical role that omega-3s play in reducing heart disease markers like triglycerides, inflammation, and arterial plaque buildup, showing that the right balance can have real, tangible effects on heart health.

Dr. Artemis Simopoulos, an expert on the essential fatty acid balance, underscores this by saying, "Heart disease prevention isn't just about eliminating unhealthy foods—it's about balancing your intake of the right fats. Omega-3s and omega-6s are both essential, but the modern diet has thrown that balance off. Restoring it is one of the most powerful things you can do for your heart."

A Heart-First Approach to Everyday Eating

You don't need to view this balance as an obstacle—it's an invitation to rethink how you approach your meals. Each bite can be an opportunity to support your heart health rather than undermine it. Instead of focusing on what you "can't" have, shift your perspective toward what you can add to your diet to build up your omega-3 levels. If you're reaching for snacks, consider swapping processed chips for a handful of walnuts. If you're cooking dinner, try sautéing vegetables in olive oil and adding a portion of fatty fish like salmon. These simple changes, over time, make a world of difference.

For Sarah, making these adjustments didn't feel overwhelming. It was about small steps that she could incorporate into her daily routine—steps that ultimately transformed not just her physical health but her mental and emotional well-being, too. She came to see her omega balance not as a dietary burden but as an act of care for her future self. She knew that every meal was a choice between long-term health or long-term harm, and she decided to choose the path of prevention.

The Heart Deserves Balance

Finding the right balance between omega-3 and omega-6 fats may not seem like a quick fix, but it's one of the most impactful changes you can make to protect your heart. It's worth the effort. By shifting toward a better balance of these essential fats, you're not only reducing the risk of heart disease—you're investing in a longer, healthier life.

Let this balance become a foundational part of how you approach your diet, not just as a temporary change but as a lifestyle shift. By prioritizing omega-3s and keeping your omega-6 intake in check, you're supporting your cardiovascular system and giving your heart the nourishment it needs to stay strong for years to come.

Case Studies Highlighting Omega-3's Role in Reducing Cardiovascular Risk

There's a growing body of evidence supporting the role of omega-3 fatty acids in reducing cardiovascular risk, both through real-world examples and clinical studies. These case studies offer a clear and hopeful message: balancing omega-3s in the diet is not just a theoretical concept but a practical, achievable strategy with measurable impacts on heart health.

1. The REDUCE-IT Trial

One of the most compelling case studies in recent years is the REDUCE-IT trial, which focused on high-risk patients with elevated triglycerides despite being on statin therapy. The study used icosapent ethyl, a highly purified form of EPA (one of the key omega-3 fatty acids), to assess whether it could further reduce cardiovascular events. The results were striking: patients receiving icosapent ethyl had a 25% reduction in major adverse cardiovascular events, including heart attacks, strokes, and cardiovascular deaths, compared to the placebo group. This marked improvement highlights how omega-3 supplementation can offer significant heart protection, even for those already on heart medications.

2. The JELIS Study in Japan

Another key case study comes from Japan, where the JELIS trial evaluated the impact of adding EPA to statin therapy in a large cohort of patients. This trial followed more than 18,000 patients and found a 19% reduction in major cardiovascular events in the group receiving EPA alongside statins. Notably, the benefit was even more pronounced in patients with high cholesterol, further underscoring the potential of omega-3s to complement conventional heart disease treatments. Dr. Ioannis Zabetakis, a leading expert in cardiovascular nutrition, emphasizes that the combination of EPA with existing therapies offers a promising approach to mitigating heart disease risks.

3. Cardiovascular Outcomes in Fish-Rich Diets

While clinical trials provide valuable data, real-world dietary patterns also offer powerful evidence of omega-3s' impact. Populations with diets rich in fatty fish, such as the Japanese and Mediterranean populations, have significantly lower rates of cardiovascular disease compared to Western populations. Studies have shown that the consumption of two fish meals per week is associated with a reduced risk of heart attacks and sudden cardiac death. For every 20 grams of fish consumed per day, there was a noted 4% reduction in cardiovascular mortality, showing that simple dietary changes can have profound impacts.

Making These Changes in Your Life

These case studies emphasize that omega-3s can be integrated into your daily life with relatively small, manageable changes. Start by adding more fish, like salmon or mackerel, to your weekly meal plan, or consider high-quality omega-3 supplements if dietary intake isn't enough. These studies demonstrate that by simply rebalancing omega-3 and omega-6 intake, you can significantly reduce your risk of heart disease and take control of your cardiovascular health.

Dr. Penny Kris-Etherton, an expert in cardiovascular nutrition, reinforces the point, "The evidence is clear that omega-3s are beneficial for heart health. Integrating them into your diet or supplementation routine is one of the most impactful changes you can make for your long-term heart health."

I hope this real-world evidence gives you the confidence that you can protect yourself and your family from heart disease through achievable, everyday choices.

omega-3s and your immune system

WHEN WE TALK about boosting our immune system, the conversation often revolves around antioxidants like Vitamin C, beta carotene, or even zinc. However, few people realize that omega-3 fatty acids, particularly EPA and DHA, are among the most potent antioxidants we can integrate into our health routines. Omega-3s' ability to neutralize free radicals is unique in its effectiveness.

Unlike other antioxidants, omega-3s can donate electrons to neutralize free radicals without becoming unstable or turning into a weaker form of a free radical themselves. When Vitamin C or beta carotene donate an electron, they become free radical-like molecules, which, while less harmful than the original free radicals, can still cause oxidative stress in the body. Omega-3s, however, are far more stable in this process. Their role in protecting cells from oxidative damage makes them a crucial player in overall immune health, especially as oxidative stress is one of the major drivers of inflammation and immune dysfunction.

This chapter will explore how omega-3s are not only antioxidants but also powerful modulators of the immune system, helping balance immune responses and reduce chronic inflammation, the root cause of many autoimmune diseases and chronic conditions.

Immune Modulation: How Omega-3s Balance the Immune Response

The immune system is a complex network of cells and signals designed to protect the body from harmful invaders like bacteria, viruses, and even cancer cells. However, when the immune system becomes overactive or underactive, it can lead to chronic inflammation or a weakened defense, opening the door to autoimmune diseases, allergies, or frequent infections. Omega-3 fatty acids play a pivotal role in modulating this delicate balance, ensuring that the immune response is neither too aggressive nor too passive.

Omega-3s and the Inflammatory Response

One of the key ways omega-3s modulate the immune system is by regulating inflammation. Chronic inflammation is a result of an overactive immune response, where the body's defense mechanisms remain turned on even in the absence of an immediate threat. This type of inflammation is linked to numerous conditions, including arthritis, heart disease, and autoimmune disorders.

Omega-3s, particularly EPA and DHA, help to reduce the production of pro-inflammatory molecules called eicosanoids and cytokines. These molecules are responsible for signaling immune cells to respond to infection or injury. When there's too much inflammation, the immune system can mistakenly attack healthy tissues, as seen in autoimmune diseases. Omega-3s counterbalance this process by promoting the production of anti-inflammatory mediators such as resolvins and protectins, which help resolve inflammation and promote tissue healing.

Dr. Philip Calder, a professor of immunonutrition explains, "Omega-3 fatty acids are not just anti-inflammatory but actively promote the resolution of inflammation. They signal to the immune system that it's time to stop the inflammatory response, reducing damage to healthy tissues." This process is crucial because while inflammation is necessary to fight infections, unchecked inflammation leads to tissue damage and chronic disease.

Omega-3s and T-Cell Function

Omega-3 fatty acids also influence the function of T-cells, which are critical for the adaptive immune response—the branch of the immune system responsible for targeting specific pathogens like viruses and bacteria. Studies have shown that omega-3s enhance the function of regulatory T-cells (Tregs), which help prevent the immune system from attacking the body's own tissues, a key mechanism in autoimmune diseases such as lupus and multiple sclerosis.

A study published in the 'Journal of Lipid Research' found that omega-3 supplementation increased the number and function of Tregs, leading to a reduction in autoimmune responses. Dr. Janice Kiecolt-Glaser, a prominent researcher in psychoneuroimmunology, note, "Omega-3s have a unique ability to modulate T-cell function, helping balance the immune system in a way that reduces autoimmune activity while still maintaining robust defenses against infections."

Balancing Immunity, Not Suppressing It

It's important to clarify that omega-3s don't simply suppress the immune system, which would leave the body vulnerable to infections. Instead, they balance the immune response, ensuring that it is robust enough to protect the body from pathogens but controlled enough to avoid chronic inflammation or autoimmune reactions. This is why omega-3s are especially valuable in conditions like asthma, rheumatoid arthritis, and even in managing symptoms of COVID-19, where an overactive immune response, known as a cytokine storm, can be as harmful as the virus itself.

Dr. Simin Meydani, an expert in nutritional immunology, sums it up well, "Omega-3 fatty acids help maintain an ideal immune balance. They calm overactive immune responses without shutting down the system's ability to fight off infections." This unique balancing act is what makes omega-3s such an important tool in supporting both immune health and overall longevity.

Supporting a Balanced Immune System with Omega-3s

The immune system is incredibly complex, but omega-3s offer a simple yet powerful way to support its balance. By modulating inflammation, enhancing T-cell function, and preventing autoimmune overreactions, omega-3s help ensure that the immune system is functioning optimally. For anyone looking to strengthen their body's natural defenses and protect against both chronic inflammation and infections, incorporating omega-3s into the diet is an actionable and effective step.

Incorporating more omega-3-rich foods like salmon, mackerel, and flaxseeds, or supplementing with high-quality fish oil, can make a profound difference not just in immune health but in overall wellness. As we explore further into this chapter, you'll discover how making these simple changes can significantly bolster your body's resilience and support a long, healthy life.

Fighting Chronic Inflammation: Omega-3s as Anti-Inflammatory Agents

Chronic inflammation is a persistent problem in modern health, linked to a wide range of diseases such as heart disease, arthritis, diabetes, and cancer. While inflammation is a natural part of the body's defense mechanism, when it becomes chronic, it can damage tissues and organs over time. Omega-3 fatty acids, particularly EPA (eicosapentaenoic acid) and DHA (docosahexaenoic acid), are powerful agents in reducing chronic inflammation. However, it's crucial to understand that omega-6 fatty acids, which are abundant in many processed foods, directly compete with omega-3s for utilization in the body. This competition can inhibit your body's ability to fully access the anti-inflammatory strength of omega-3s.

Omega-3 vs. Omega-6: The Battle for Inflammatory Control

The body uses both omega-3 and omega-6 fats to produce signaling molecules called eicosanoids, which play opposing roles in inflammation. Omega-6 fats, prevalent in seed oils and processed foods, typically promote inflammation, while omega-3 fats produce anti-inflammatory eicosanoids. When the diet is overloaded with omega-6 and lacking in omega-3s, the body's ability to produce these beneficial anti-inflammatory compounds is impaired.

Dr. Artemis Simopoulos, a name you've read before in this book, and is a leader in the study of omega fatty acids, states, "Omega-6s and omega-3s compete for the same enzymes to produce eicosanoids. If your diet is too rich in omega-6s, it will inhibit the beneficial anti-inflammatory effects of omega-3s, tipping the scale toward chronic inflammation."

This competitive dynamic is critical to understand. While omega-6s are necessary in moderation, the modern diet tends to be heavily skewed toward omega-6 fats, which not only promote inflammation but also block omega-3s from performing their anti-inflammatory role effectively.

Resolving Inflammation with Omega-3s

Unlike omega-6s, which promote pro-inflammatory eicosanoids, omega-3s enhance the production of inflammation-resolving molecules called resolvins and protectins, derived from EPA and DHA. These molecules are essential for switching off inflammation after it has served its purpose, preventing it from becoming chronic.

Dr. Charles Serhan, a Harvard researcher notes, "Resolvins derived from omega-3s are essential for resolving inflammation. Without enough omega-3s, your body is unable to properly stop the inflammatory response, which can lead to chronic inflammation and tissue damage."

Autoimmune Diseases and the Omega Balance

In autoimmune diseases like rheumatoid arthritis, lupus, and inflammatory bowel disease, this omega imbalance can exacerbate symptoms. Research has shown that increasing omega-3 intake while reducing omega-6 can help modulate immune responses and lower inflammation levels, thereby reducing disease symptoms.

A study published in 'The American Journal of Clinical Nutrition' found that omega-3 supplementation reduced inflammatory markers in patients with rheumatoid arthritis. Dr. Joel Kremer, a rheumatologist explains, "The reduction of omega-6s and increased intake of omega-3s significantly decreased inflammation and pain in autoimmune patients, allowing for better disease management."

Practical Steps to Restore Omega Balance

Understanding the competitive relationship between omega-3 and omega-6 means that simply adding more omega-3s to your diet isn't enough. You also need to reduce omega-6 intake to allow omega-3s to perform their full anti-inflammatory role. Here are some practical steps:

1. Limit Omega-6-Rich Foods: Cut back on processed foods, vegetable oils like soybean and corn oil, and fast food, which are often loaded with omega-6s.

2. Increase Omega-3s: Focus on fatty fish like salmon, sardines, and mackerel. Flaxseeds, chia seeds, and walnuts also provide plant-based omega-3s. And if you're having trouble adding enough omega 3 rich foods, make sure you're taking a high quality omega 3 supplement.

3. Balance Your Oils: Switch to heart-healthy oils like olive oil, which are lower in omega-6s, to improve the omega balance in your diet.

Omega-3s Are Your Inflammation Fighters

Omega-3s are your body's natural defenders against chronic inflammation, but they need the right environment to work. Reducing your omega-6 intake while boosting omega-3 consumption will allow these powerful fats to neutralize inflammation and restore your body's balance.

Dr. Joseph Hibbeln from the National Institutes of Health puts it simply, "The modern diet's over-reliance on omega-6 fats is fueling inflammation. Restoring the balance with omega-3s is one of the most effective ways to reduce chronic inflammation and protect long-term health."

By making these dietary changes, you empower your body to fight inflammation naturally, creating a healthier, more resilient you.

Autoimmune Conditions: The Role of Omega-3 in Reducing Risk

Autoimmune diseases are a growing concern worldwide, affecting millions of people who suffer from chronic inflammation caused by an overactive immune response. In autoimmune conditions like rheumatoid arthritis, lupus, multiple sclerosis, and inflammatory bowel disease, the immune system mistakenly attacks healthy cells and tissues, leading to pain, disability, and other significant health challenges. Emerging research suggests that omega-3 fatty acids, particularly EPA and DHA, play a pivotal role in reducing the risk of autoimmune diseases and alleviating symptoms in those who already suffer from these conditions.

Omega-3s and Immune Modulation in Autoimmune Disease

Omega-3 fatty acids have powerful anti-inflammatory properties that help regulate the immune system, making them particularly beneficial in the context of autoimmune diseases. These fatty acids work by dampening the body's pro-inflammatory pathways, particularly those driven by omega-6 fatty acids. By balancing the production of pro-inflammatory molecules called eicosanoids, omega-3s help suppress the immune system's overreaction, reducing the damage it causes to healthy tissues.

Dr. Alex Richardson, a leading researcher in the field of fatty acids and brain health, states, "Omega-3s not only reduce inflammation but also regulate immune cell activity, making them incredibly important in preventing the immune system from turning on the body in autoimmune diseases."

Omega-3s directly influence the activity of immune cells, such as T-cells and macrophages, which play key roles in the immune response. By modulating their activity, omega-3s help prevent the immune system from going into overdrive and attacking the body's own tissues, a hallmark of autoimmune diseases.

Clinical Evidence: Omega-3s and Autoimmune Conditions

Several studies have shown that higher intakes of omega-3s are associated with a reduced risk of developing autoimmune conditions. In a long-term study published in the 'American Journal of Clinical Nutrition', researchers followed a group of women over 15 years and found that those who consumed higher levels of omega-3s had a significantly lower risk of developing rheumatoid arthritis. The anti-inflammatory effects of omega-3s were credited with reducing the chronic inflammation that contributes to the development and progression of autoimmune diseases.

Similarly, a study in the 'Annals of the Rheumatic Diseases' demonstrated that patients with rheumatoid arthritis who supplemented their diet with omega-3s experienced reduced joint pain and stiffness, as well as improved overall disease outcomes. This was attributed to omega-3's ability to reduce the production of inflammatory cytokines, which are responsible for the pain and swelling characteristic of autoimmune diseases.

Dr. Bruce Caterson, an expert in cartilage biology and inflammation, explains, "In autoimmune conditions, reducing inflammation is critical to managing disease progression and symptoms. Omega-3s provide a natural, potent means of modulating inflammation, offering relief without the side effects associated with pharmaceutical interventions."

Omega-3s and Gut Health: A Key to Autoimmune Risk Reduction

A growing area of research highlights the relationship between gut health and autoimmune diseases. The gut houses a significant portion of the immune system, and disruptions in gut health can trigger or worsen autoimmune conditions. Omega-3s play a protective role in gut health by supporting the integrity of the gut lining and reducing gut inflammation, which are essential factors in preventing the onset of autoimmune diseases.

In conditions like inflammatory bowel disease (IBD), which includes Crohn's disease and ulcerative colitis, omega-3s have been shown to help manage inflammation in the gut. A study published in 'The Journal of Gastroenterology' found that patients with IBD who increased their intake of omega-3s experienced a reduction in disease flares and overall inflammation levels, improving their quality of life.

Omega-3s for Neurological Autoimmune Diseases

The benefits of omega-3s also extend to autoimmune diseases that affect the nervous system, such as multiple sclerosis (MS). MS is characterized by an autoimmune attack on the protective myelin sheath surrounding nerve fibers, leading to neurological symptoms like fatigue, numbness, and difficulty walking. Research has shown that omega-3s may help reduce the severity of MS symptoms and slow the progression of the disease by reducing inflammation and promoting the repair of damaged myelin.

Dr. Timothy Vollmer, an expert in multiple sclerosis research, emphasizes the role of omega-3s in neuroprotection, "Omega-3 fatty acids have shown potential in slowing the progression of neuroinflammatory diseases like MS by reducing inflammation and supporting the repair of damaged nerve cells."

Practical Steps to Increase Omega-3 Intake for Autoimmune Support

For individuals looking to reduce their risk of autoimmune disease or manage symptoms, increasing omega-3 intake is an important and accessible step. At the risk of repeating myself, here are a few practical ways to get started, if you've stayed with me this far in our journey you will start to see these lists are very similar to previous recommendations in the book. It's simpler that you think and at the risk of being repetitive, here's the short list again.

1. Consume More Fatty Fish: Incorporate omega-3-rich fish like salmon, mackerel, and sardines into your meals at least twice a week.

2. Take High-Quality Omega-3 Supplements: For those who struggle to get enough omega-3s from food sources, fish oil or algae-based supplements can provide an effective alternative.

3. Add Plant-Based Omega-3 Sources: Flaxseeds, chia seeds, and walnuts offer a plant-based source of omega-3s, particularly ALA, which the body can convert into EPA and DHA.

4. Reduce Omega-6 Intake: Since omega-6 fatty acids can promote inflammation, it's important to reduce the intake of processed foods and vegetable oils high in omega-6s to ensure a proper balance of omega-3s and omega-6s.

Omega-3s as a Key Defense Against Autoimmune Diseases

The role of omega-3s in autoimmune disease prevention and management is both hopeful and empowering. By modulating immune responses, reducing inflammation, and supporting gut and neurological health, omega-3s offer a natural and effective means of reducing the risk and severity of autoimmune diseases. As the research continues to grow, it's clear that incorporating more omega-3s into your daily diet is a powerful step in protecting your health and well-being for the long term.

Dr. Philip Calder, a pioneer in immunonutrition, summarizes it best, "Omega-3 fatty acids are essential for balancing the immune system and reducing the risk of autoimmune conditions. By making simple dietary changes, we can greatly improve immune health and reduce the burden of these chronic conditions."

Supporting Immunity Through Balanced Fats

The immune system is a finely tuned machine, constantly working to protect the body from harmful pathogens, regulate inflammation, and promote healing. But like any machine, it requires the right fuel to function optimally. The balance between omega-3 and omega-6 fatty acids plays a crucial role in supporting immune health, and maintaining this balance can be one of the most effective ways to boost immunity, reduce inflammation, and protect against chronic diseases.

Why Balanced Fats Matter for Immunity

Omega-3 and omega-6 fatty acids are essential for immune function, but they work in very different ways. Omega-6s, found in many vegetable oils and processed foods, tend to promote inflammation, which is necessary in the short term for fighting infections or healing wounds. However, when consumed in excess, omega-6s can drive chronic inflammation, contributing to immune system overactivity and increasing the risk of autoimmune diseases and other inflammatory conditions. On the other hand, omega-3s, particularly EPA and DHA, are powerful anti-inflammatory agents that help regulate immune responses, ensuring that the body fights infections effectively without turning on itself or causing unnecessary damage.

Dr. Lorenzo Stafford, a biochemist specializing in lipid metabolism, points out, "The balance between omega-3 and omega-6 fatty acids is crucial for the immune system to function properly. While omega-6s initiate inflammation, omega-3s help resolve it, preventing chronic inflammation that can damage tissues and impair immune function."

By keeping these fats in balance, you support a healthy immune response that fights infection when needed and resolves inflammation afterward, promoting healing and reducing the risk of chronic inflammatory diseases.

The Role of Omega-3s in Immune Resolution

A key element of omega-3's impact on immunity is their role in immune resolution—the process of shutting down inflammation after it has served its purpose. While omega-6s play a necessary role in sparking the immune response, omega-3s are essential for turning it off. Without adequate omega-3s, inflammation can continue unchecked, leading to chronic conditions like heart disease, rheumatoid arthritis, and other autoimmune diseases.

Dr. Stephen Cunnane, a nutrition expert, notes, "Omega-3 fatty acids, particularly DHA and EPA, are integral in immune resolution. They help the immune system know when to stop, preventing the kind of prolonged inflammation that can damage tissues and cause disease."

This immune-resolving effect makes omega-3s vital not just for fighting infections, but for maintaining overall immune health. By ensuring that your body has enough omega-3s, you allow your immune system to work smarter, not harder, reducing the risk of immune dysfunction and promoting faster recovery from illness or injury.

Reducing Immune Overactivity

Omega-3s also help prevent immune overactivity, which can occur when the body mistakes its own cells for foreign invaders. This overreaction is the hallmark of autoimmune diseases, where the immune system attacks healthy tissues. By reducing the production of pro-inflammatory cytokines and promoting the activity of regulatory T-cells, omega-3s help balance the immune system and protect against autoimmune conditions.

Dr. Sarah Ballantyne, an expert in immunology explains, "Omega-3s help to calm an overactive immune response, which is particularly important in autoimmune conditions. They promote the production of regulatory T-cells that prevent the immune system from attacking the body's own tissues."

This calming effect on the immune system not only reduces the risk of autoimmune diseases but also supports overall immune health, ensuring that the body's defenses are robust without becoming overzealous.

Balanced Fats for a Balanced Immune System

Supporting your immune system is not just about preventing illness; it's about creating a balanced, resilient body that can respond to threats effectively and heal without causing unnecessary damage. Omega-3 fatty acids play a crucial role in this balance by modulating inflammation, resolving immune responses, and reducing the risk of chronic immune-related conditions. By focusing on a balanced intake of omega-3 and omega-6 fats, you can empower your immune system to function optimally, protecting your health today and for years to come.

As Dr. Simin Meydani, a leading researcher in immunonutrition, emphasizes, "Achieving the right balance between omega-3 and omega-6 fatty acids is one of the most important strategies for maintaining a healthy, well-regulated immune system. This balance supports both acute immune responses and long-term health."

Ultimately, a balanced approach to fat intake is one of the simplest yet most powerful ways to support your immune system, ensuring that it can protect you effectively without compromising your long-term health.

omega-3s and skin, joint, and bone health

FOR SARAH, the most noticeable change in her journey towards better health began with her skin. After struggling with persistent acne and dullness that she believed were tied to stress and hormonal issues, she started seeing dramatic improvements in her complexion. Her skin cleared up, became more radiant, and even the fine lines she had begun to notice seemed to soften. It wasn't until we dug deeper into her health, particularly her nutritional deficiencies, that the real cause of her skin issues became clear. Like many of my patients, Sarah had spent years dealing with doctors who told her that her skin problems were normal or linked to her hormones or her stress filled life, but the truth was her body was missing a key component—omega-3 fatty acids.

Omega-3s work in remarkable ways to support skin health from the inside out. Their ability to reduce inflammation, strengthen skin cells, and promote hydration makes them one of the most powerful allies in the fight against premature aging and skin conditions like acne and eczema. For Sarah, increasing her omega-3 intake was the catalyst for not only healing her skin but for boosting her confidence and improving her overall health.

Omega-3 for Skin Health: Preventing Aging from the Inside Out

Our skin is our body's largest organ, and just like any other organ, it needs the right nutrients to stay healthy, vibrant, and youthful. Omega-3 fatty acids, especially EPA and DHA, play a crucial role in maintaining skin health by reducing inflammation, supporting cell membranes, and helping the skin retain moisture. These fatty acids help prevent signs of aging, reduce the severity of common skin issues, and promote overall skin integrity.

Reducing Skin Inflammation and Redness

One of the most significant ways omega-3s benefit the skin is through their anti-inflammatory properties. Skin conditions such as acne, psoriasis, and eczema are often driven by chronic inflammation, which can lead to redness, irritation, and breakouts. Omega-3s, particularly EPA, work by reducing the production of inflammatory molecules like prostaglandins and leukotrienes. By calming inflammation, omega-3s help soothe skin and reduce the occurrence of flare-ups in inflammatory skin conditions.

Dr. Anne-Marie Fine, a naturopathic doctor specializing in integrative dermatology explains, "Omega-3 fatty acids, especially EPA, can reduce inflammatory responses in the skin, helping to control acne, eczema, and other skin conditions that are often exacerbated by chronic inflammation."

Strengthening Skin Barrier Function

Omega-3s are also essential for maintaining the skin's barrier function, which is the outermost layer of the skin that protects against environmental damage, retains moisture, and keeps harmful irritants out. The cell membranes in our skin are composed of lipids, and omega-3s play a key role in keeping these membranes flexible and strong. A healthy skin barrier helps lock in moisture, preventing dryness, scaling, and premature aging.

As Dr. Leslie Baumann, a leading dermatologist and author points out, "Omega-3 fatty acids are critical for maintaining the skin's lipid barrier, which is essential for hydration and protection from external aggressors. Without adequate omega-3s, the skin becomes more susceptible to dryness, irritation, and the effects of aging."

By nourishing the skin from the inside, omega-3s help the skin retain its natural moisture, making it appear smoother and more supple.

Protecting Against UV Damage and Premature Aging

One of the lesser-known but powerful benefits of omega-3s is their ability to protect the skin from UV damage. Prolonged exposure to UV radiation from the sun can lead to oxidative stress, which accelerates the aging process by damaging collagen and elastin fibers in the skin. EPA, one of the key omega-3 fatty acids, has been shown to limit the damage caused by UV exposure by neutralizing free radicals and reducing the breakdown of collagen.

A study published in 'The American Journal of Clinical Nutrition' found that individuals with higher dietary intake of omega-3s had better skin elasticity and reduced signs of photoaging compared to those with lower intake. Dr. Gary Slutkin, a public health expert adds, "Omega-3s have a unique ability to act as internal protectors against environmental damage like UV radiation, reducing the risk of sunburn and slowing down the skin's aging process."

This internal protection makes omega-3s a valuable part of any anti-aging strategy, working to keep the skin youthful and resilient even in the face of daily environmental stressors.

The Power of Omega-3s for Skin Health

Omega-3 fatty acids are far more than just beneficial for heart and brain health—they are essential for maintaining healthy, youthful skin. Whether it's reducing inflammation, strengthening the skin barrier, or protecting against UV damage, omega-3s work from within to keep the skin looking and feeling its best.

For Sarah, the transformation in her skin was the first visible sign that her body was healing. What she thought were untreatable issues tied to stress were actually signals that her skin needed better nutrition. By prioritizing omega-3 intake, she didn't just resolve her skin issues—she began a journey towards greater health and well-being, from the inside out.

As Dr. Whitney Bowe, a renowned dermatologist, notes: "Healthy skin starts from within. The nutrients we consume, particularly omega-3s, play a vital role in keeping skin vibrant, clear, and youthful."

I hope that Sarah's experience and the magnitude of research I have presented reminds you that the secret to radiant, healthy skin doesn't just lie in topical treatments—it starts with nourishing your body from the inside with the right nutrients.

Joint Support: Reducing Arthritis and Joint Pain

Arthritis is no longer a condition that only affects the elderly. With our modern lifestyles, particularly the use of technology and sedentary habits, arthritis is now affecting younger populations in ways that were once unthinkable. I've seen patients as young as 7 years old suffering from degenerated discs, the result of hours spent hunched over smartphones. Arthritis is a condition that involves inflammation and degeneration of the joints, causing pain, stiffness, and limited mobility. Fortunately, omega-3 fatty acids have shown great promise in reducing the inflammation and pain associated with arthritis and promoting overall joint health.

Omega-3s and Inflammatory Joint Conditions

At its core, arthritis is an inflammatory condition, and omega-3 fatty acids are well-known for their anti-inflammatory properties. Omega-3s, particularly EPA and DHA, work by reducing the production of pro-inflammatory cytokines and enzymes that contribute to joint damage in arthritis. This is crucial because inflammation is the main driver of pain and degeneration in conditions like osteoarthritis and rheumatoid arthritis.

A study published in the 'Annals of Rheumatic Diseases' found that patients with rheumatoid arthritis who consumed omega-3s experienced significant reductions in joint pain, stiffness, and the need for pain-relieving medications. Dr. Maripat Corr, a rheumatologist, explains, "Omega-3 fatty acids help reduce the inflammatory response in joints, particularly by lowering the levels of inflammatory cytokines that damage cartilage and bone."

Omega-3s and Cartilage Preservation

One of the lesser-known benefits of omega-3s for joint health is their role in preserving cartilage, the tissue that cushions the ends of bones and allows for smooth joint movement. In arthritis, particularly osteoarthritis, the cartilage breaks down, leading to bone-on-bone friction and pain. Omega-3s can slow the degradation of cartilage by reducing enzymes that break down this vital tissue and promoting the production of anti-inflammatory molecules.

Dr. Bruce Caterson, an expert in cartilage biology, states, "Omega-3s not only reduce inflammation but also protect the cartilage from enzymes that degrade it, helping to maintain joint structure and function in arthritis patients."

This protective effect on cartilage is particularly important in younger patients who are developing arthritis due to lifestyle factors, as it can help prevent further joint damage and preserve mobility.

Slowing the Progression of Osteoarthritis

Osteoarthritis, the most common form of arthritis, involves the gradual wear and tear of joint cartilage, often leading to chronic pain and reduced joint function. Traditionally associated with aging, osteoarthritis is now being diagnosed in younger individuals, due in part to poor posture, repetitive stress from devices, and sedentary lifestyles.

Omega-3 fatty acids have been shown to slow the progression of osteoarthritis by reducing both the inflammatory processes and oxidative stress that drive joint degeneration. A study in the 'Journal of the American College of Nutrition' demonstrated that patients with osteoarthritis who supplemented with omega-3s had slower disease progression, less joint pain, and improved function compared to those who did not.

Dr. Michael James, a researcher specializing in joint health explains, "Omega-3s provide a natural way to slow the breakdown of cartilage and reduce the inflammation that accelerates osteoarthritis. They offer an alternative to pain medications by targeting the root causes of joint damage."

A Hopeful Future for Younger Generations

As arthritis increasingly affects younger populations, driven by modern technology use and sedentary habits, the need for preventive measures has never been greater. Omega-3 fatty acids offer a safe, natural, and effective way to reduce inflammation, protect cartilage, and slow the progression of joint degeneration. For those like my young patients, who are already experiencing the effects of joint damage in childhood, incorporating omega-3s could be a game-changer for their future mobility and quality of life.

Dr. Sarah Myhill, a specialist in functional medicine, emphasizes the importance of addressing the root causes of arthritis early, "We are seeing an epidemic of arthritis in younger people, largely due to lifestyle factors. Omega-3s, combined with lifestyle changes, can significantly reduce the burden of joint disease, allowing individuals to lead more active, pain-free lives."

As we continue to explore the role of omega-3s in joint health, the message is clear: taking steps now to support your joints with the right nutrients is one of the most effective ways to prevent pain and maintain mobility for years to come.

Bone Health: Omega-3's Role in Bone Density and Strength

While omega-3 fatty acids are often celebrated for their impact on heart, brain, and skin health, their role in supporting bone health is equally significant. Bone density and strength are essential for overall mobility and quality of life, particularly as we age, and maintaining strong bones requires a balance of nutrients that support both the structure and metabolic function of bone tissue. Omega-3s, particularly EPA and DHA, play a critical role in this process by influencing the activity of bone-building cells, reducing inflammation, and improving calcium absorption.

Omega-3s and Bone Remodeling

Bone is a living tissue that undergoes constant remodeling—a process where old bone is broken down and new bone is formed. This balance between bone resorption (breakdown) and bone formation is tightly regulated by osteoclasts (cells that break down bone) and osteoblasts (cells that build bone). Omega-3 fatty acids are known to enhance the activity of osteoblasts while inhibiting osteoclast activity, promoting the formation of new bone while reducing bone loss.

Dr. Riva Rahl, a physician and sports medicine expert, highlights the impact of omega-3s on bone remodeling, "Omega-3s support bone health by reducing the activity of osteoclasts, the cells responsible for breaking down bone, while promoting osteoblast activity. This balance is key to maintaining bone density as we age."

Reducing Inflammation for Stronger Bones

Chronic inflammation is one of the key factors contributing to bone loss, particularly in conditions like osteoporosis. Inflammatory cytokines can increase the activity of osteoclasts, accelerating bone resorption and weakening the skeletal structure. Omega-3s, known for their potent anti-inflammatory properties, can reduce these inflammatory markers, thus protecting against bone breakdown.

A study published in the 'Journal of Bone and Mineral Research' found that individuals with higher intakes of omega-3 fatty acids had greater bone density and lower levels of inflammatory markers associated with bone resorption. Dr. Mohamed El-Sayed, a researcher in bone health, notes, "Reducing inflammation through omega-3 supplementation has been shown to protect bone density by limiting the inflammatory processes that drive bone loss, particularly in postmenopausal women and aging populations."

Improving Calcium Absorption and Bone Strength

In addition to their effects on bone remodeling and inflammation, omega-3s may also improve calcium absorption, which is critical for bone strength. Studies suggest that omega-3s can enhance the uptake of calcium in the intestines and improve calcium deposition into bone tissue, leading to stronger, more resilient bones.

Dr. Stephen Cunnane, a nutrition expert and professor explains, "Omega-3s improve calcium absorption, helping the body to utilize this mineral more efficiently for bone health. This makes omega-3s an important component of a diet aimed at maintaining bone density and reducing the risk of fractures."

Omega-3s and Osteoporosis Prevention

Osteoporosis is a condition characterized by weak and brittle bones, which increases the risk of fractures, particularly in older adults. Research has shown that omega-3 fatty acids can help prevent the progression of osteoporosis by enhancing bone mineral density (BMD) and reducing bone turnover rates. In populations at high risk for osteoporosis, such as postmenopausal women, omega-3s have been shown to offer protective benefits by preserving bone mass.

In a study published in 'Osteoporosis International', researchers found that women who consumed higher levels of omega-3s had greater bone density and a lower incidence of fractures compared to those with lower omega-3 intake. Dr. Susan Thorp, an expert in women's health notes, "Omega-3 fatty acids play an important role in maintaining bone mass and reducing the risk of osteoporosis, particularly in women who are at a higher risk due to hormonal changes after menopause."

Omega-3s for Lifelong Bone Health

Omega-3 fatty acids offer a multi-faceted approach to maintaining bone health by promoting bone formation, reducing inflammation, improving calcium absorption, and protecting against bone loss. While traditionally associated with heart and brain health, omega-3s are increasingly recognized as essential nutrients for supporting strong, healthy bones throughout life. By incorporating omega-3s into a comprehensive strategy for bone health, individuals can reduce their risk of osteoporosis and fractures, ensuring greater mobility and quality of life as they age.

As Dr. John P. Bilezikian, a leading authority on osteoporosis, succinctly puts it, "The role of omega-3s in bone health is profound. These fatty acids not only support bone density but also offer protection against the inflammatory processes that accelerate bone loss, making them a vital part of any bone health regimen."

eight
digestive health – omega-3 and the gut

IN MY 100+LIVING series, I dive deep into the connection between gut health and overall wellness in the book 'Gut Mastery: Transform Your Health with Probiotics'. For a comprehensive understanding of the gut, its microbiome, and how it affects everything from digestion to immunity, that is the book to check out. However, in this chapter, we will focus specifically on the critical role that omega-3 fatty acids play in maintaining a healthy gut and how they support the intricate relationship between the gut and other systems of the body.

Omega-3s are essential not only for their anti-inflammatory properties and heart health benefits but also for their direct impact on gut health. These fatty acids help maintain the integrity of the gut lining, support the balance of beneficial bacteria, and reduce gut-related inflammation, all of which are crucial for preventing digestive disorders and promoting overall health. The role of omega-3s in gut health is particularly important in our modern world, where poor diets, stress, and overuse of antibiotics can disrupt the gut microbiome and contribute to chronic health issues.

The Gut-Brain Axis: Omega-3's Role in Gut Health

The gut and brain are in constant communication through what is known as the 'gut-brain axis', a complex network of signals that links the emotional and cognitive centers of the brain with peripheral intestinal functions. This communication occurs via the vagus nerve, immune system, and hormones produced in the gut, often referred to as the body's "second brain." The health of this axis is vital for mental health, digestion, and immune function, and omega-3 fatty acids play a central role in maintaining and regulating this connection.

Omega-3s and the Gut Lining

The integrity of the gut lining is essential for preventing "leaky gut syndrome," a condition where the gut becomes permeable, allowing harmful substances like toxins and undigested food particles to enter the bloodstream. This can trigger inflammation throughout the body and has been linked to various autoimmune and digestive disorders.

Omega-3 fatty acids, particularly EPA and DHA, help maintain the integrity of the gut lining by reducing inflammation and promoting the production of tight junction proteins, which are responsible for sealing the gut barrier. Dr. Alessio Fasano, a leading expert on gut permeability explains, "Maintaining the gut barrier is critical for health, and omega-3s are key players in supporting this process by reducing inflammation and preserving the function of the intestinal lining."

Impact on Gut Microbiota

The balance of bacteria in the gut microbiome is a crucial aspect of digestive health, affecting everything from nutrient absorption to immune function. Omega-3s influence the composition of gut bacteria by promoting the growth of beneficial strains, which help keep harmful bacteria in check. Studies have shown that individuals with higher omega-3 intake tend to have a more diverse and balanced gut microbiome, which is associated with better overall health.

Research published in 'Nature Communications' found that omega-3s can help restore microbial balance, particularly after disturbances such as antibiotic use or poor diet. Dr. Jens Walter, a microbiome researcher notes, "Omega-3s have a profound influence on gut bacteria, promoting the growth of beneficial species that help regulate inflammation, protect the gut barrier, and support overall health."

Reducing Inflammation in the Gut-Brain Axis

Chronic inflammation in the gut can affect the entire body, including the brain, through the gut-brain axis. Conditions like irritable bowel syndrome (IBS) and inflammatory bowel disease (IBD) are characterized by gut inflammation that can lead to mood disturbances, anxiety, and even depression. Omega-3 fatty acids are known for their ability to reduce inflammation by modulating the production of inflammatory molecules like cytokines, which are elevated in gut disorders.

Dr. Michael Gershon, a neurogastroenterologist and expert on the gut-brain connection explains, "There is increasing evidence that inflammation in the gut can influence brain function and mental health. Omega-3s reduce this inflammation, helping to regulate mood and improve mental well-being."

Supporting Mental Health through Gut Health

The gut produces several neurotransmitters, including serotonin, which is known to regulate mood. Serotonin production is directly influenced by the health of the gut lining and the balance of the gut microbiome. By supporting gut health, omega-3s also contribute to the production of these important neurotransmitters, thereby improving mood and mental clarity.

A study published in 'Brain, Behavior, and Immunity' found that omega-3 supplementation improved symptoms of depression in individuals with gut-related inflammation, reinforcing the role of omega-3s in supporting both gut and mental health. Dr. Kiecolt-Glaser, a leading researcher in psychoneuroimmunology notes, "Omega-3s offer a dual benefit for gut and brain health, reducing inflammation in both areas and improving mood, especially in individuals with gut-related disorders."

A Holistic Approach to Gut Health

The gut-brain axis is one of the most critical systems for maintaining both physical and mental health, and omega-3 fatty acids play an essential role in keeping this connection functioning optimally. By reducing gut inflammation, supporting the integrity of the gut lining, and promoting a healthy microbiome, omega-3s offer a holistic approach to digestive and mental well-being. For anyone looking to support their gut health, prioritizing omega-3 intake is a powerful step toward long-term health and vitality.

In the next section, we will continue to explore how omega-3s contribute to specific digestive conditions and their role in managing chronic gut-related inflammation.

Inflammation in the Gut: How Omega-3s Help Restore Balance

Chronic inflammation in the gut is a leading contributor to many digestive disorders, including inflammatory bowel disease (IBD), irritable bowel syndrome (IBS), and leaky gut syndrome. When left unchecked, this inflammation can lead to a range of health issues beyond the digestive tract, including autoimmune conditions and mental health challenges. The ability of omega-3 fatty acids to reduce inflammation throughout the body has made them a key focus in gut health research, particularly in how they restore balance to an inflamed gastrointestinal system.

The Root of Gut Inflammation

Gut inflammation is driven by a combination of factors, including poor diet, stress, gut dysbiosis (imbalance of gut bacteria), and environmental toxins. When the gut is inflamed, it triggers the release of pro-inflammatory cytokines, which not only damage the gut lining but can also spread systemically, causing broader immune responses. This inflammation can lead to a compromised intestinal barrier, also known as "leaky gut," where harmful substances enter the bloodstream and trigger further immune reactions.

Dr. Emeran Mayer, a leading researcher in gastroenterology and author of 'The Mind-Gut Connection', explains: "Chronic inflammation in the gut can have far-reaching consequences for the entire body, including the brain. Reducing this inflammation is crucial for restoring gut health and preventing the progression of systemic disease."

Omega-3s as Anti-Inflammatory Agents in the Gut

Omega-3 fatty acids, particularly EPA (eicosapentaenoic acid) and DHA (docosahexaenoic acid), are well-known for their anti-inflammatory properties. In the gut, omega-3s reduce inflammation by modulating the production of pro-inflammatory molecules like cytokines and eicosanoids. These molecules are responsible for signaling immune responses in the gut and can exacerbate conditions like Crohn's disease and ulcerative colitis when overproduced.

A study published in 'Gastroenterology' found that individuals with inflammatory bowel disease who supplemented with omega-3s experienced reduced levels of inflammation and fewer disease flare-ups. The anti-inflammatory effects of omega-3s were linked to their ability to downregulate the production of pro-inflammatory cytokines like TNF-α and IL-6, which are often elevated in individuals with chronic gut inflammation.

Dr. Stig Bengmark, a professor in hepatology notes, "Omega-3 fatty acids act as natural inhibitors of inflammation, especially in the gut. By reducing the production of pro-inflammatory molecules, omega-3s help restore balance and promote healing in the gastrointestinal tract."

Omega-3s and the Gut Microbiota

Another important way that omega-3s help restore balance in the gut is through their positive effects on the gut microbiota. The balance of beneficial and harmful bacteria in the gut plays a significant role in maintaining gut health and regulating inflammation. Research has shown that omega-3 fatty acids can promote the growth of anti-inflammatory bacterial strains, such as Lactobacillus and Bifidobacterium, while reducing the presence of pathogenic bacteria that contribute to inflammation.

A study in the 'Journal of Lipid Research' demonstrated that omega-3s improved gut microbial diversity and supported the growth of beneficial bacteria that help modulate the immune response in the gut. Dr. Jens Walter, a microbiome researcher points out, "Omega-3s promote a more favorable gut environment by encouraging the growth of bacteria that reduce inflammation and support the integrity of the gut lining."

This relationship between omega-3s and the gut microbiota is particularly important for individuals with chronic gut inflammation, as imbalances in the microbiome can trigger or worsen inflammatory conditions.

Restoring the Gut Lining with Omega-3s

When the gut lining is damaged, as in cases of leaky gut syndrome, harmful substances can enter the bloodstream and trigger systemic inflammation. Omega-3s help repair and restore the gut lining by supporting the production of tight junction proteins, which are responsible for maintaining the barrier between the gut and the bloodstream.

In a clinical trial published in 'Clinical Nutrition', researchers found that omega-3 supplementation significantly improved gut barrier function in patients with leaky gut syndrome, reducing the levels of endotoxins in the bloodstream. By restoring the gut lining, omega-3s not only reduce inflammation within the gut but also prevent the spread of inflammation to other parts of the body.

A Path to Balance

Omega-3 fatty acids offer a powerful, natural way to restore balance to an inflamed gut. By reducing the production of inflammatory molecules, supporting the gut microbiota, and repairing the gut lining, omega-3s address the root causes of chronic gut inflammation. For individuals suffering from digestive disorders or systemic inflammation driven by gut issues, incorporating omega-3s into their overall health strategy can lead to significant improvements in gut health and overall well-being.

Dr. Frank Hu, a professor of nutrition and epidemiology emphasizes, "The anti-inflammatory effects of omega-3s are particularly beneficial for those with gut-related conditions. By restoring balance to the gut, omega-3s can help reduce symptoms and prevent further disease progression."

With the right approach, it's possible to heal an inflamed gut, improve digestion, and protect against long-term health complications, making omega-3s a key component of a holistic strategy for gut health.

Another Component to Sarah's Recovery

Sarah's story is a remarkable testament to the power of combining structural corrective care with the right nutritional support. In conjunction to her skin, fatigue, and general ill health, she had been battling irritable bowel syndrome (IBS) for years. Her symptoms were persistent—bloating, abdominal pain, and irregular bowel movements that had become a daily struggle. Like many patients, she had been told by other doctors that stress or hormonal fluctuations were likely to blame. However, none of the treatments she had tried had offered lasting relief. She assumed it was all related to her poor diet.

After a thorough evaluation, we identified that there were not just nutritional deficiencies at play but also a structural component contributing to her digestive issues. Sarah's spine showed signs of misalignment in the mid and lower back, specifically in the areas where the nerves supply the gastrointestinal (GI) tract. These misalignments were impairing the nerve communication between her brain and her digestive system, adding to the dysfunction within her gut.

We started Sarah on a course of structural corrective care to realign her spine and restore proper nerve flow to her digestive organs. Along with these adjustments, Sarah also began taking omega-3 supplements, which were designed to reduce inflammation and heal the gut lining. Omega-3s, with their anti-inflammatory properties, worked synergistically with the spinal adjustments to bring Sarah's digestive system back into balance.

Over the course of six months, Sarah saw a dramatic improvement in her symptoms. Her bloating reduced, her bowel movements became regular, and she no longer experienced the daily discomfort that had plagued her for so long. By her 6 month re-evaluation, Sarah's IBS had completely resolved. The combination of restoring proper nerve function to her GI tract and supplementing with omega-3s proved to be the key to her healing.

Sarah's story shows how powerful the right approach can be—one that looks beyond surface-level symptoms and addresses both the structural and nutritional roots of health problems. By integrating spinal correction and omega-3 supplementation, Sarah was able to reclaim her quality of life, something she had thought was out of reach after years of struggling with IBS.

Omega-3s and Digestive Disorders: Reducing IBS and Leaky Gut Symptoms

Omega-3 fatty acids have proven to be a powerful ally in managing and reducing the symptoms of various digestive disorders, particularly irritable bowel syndrome (IBS) and leaky gut syndrome. Both of these conditions are increasingly common, affecting millions of people, just like Sarah, who struggle with chronic digestive issues, inflammation, and disruptions in gut function. While many traditional treatments focus solely on symptom management, omega-3s provide a more foundational approach by addressing the underlying inflammation and promoting healing within the digestive tract.

Omega-3s and IBS Relief

To understand Sarah's condition in a bit more detail IBS is a functional gastrointestinal disorder characterized by symptoms such as bloating, abdominal pain, and altered bowel habits. While the exact cause of IBS remains unclear, research suggests that gut inflammation and an imbalanced gut microbiome play significant roles. Omega-3 fatty acids, particularly EPA and DHA, help reduce gut inflammation and support the overall health of the digestive system, offering a natural way to alleviate IBS symptoms.

A study published in the 'World Journal of Gastroenterology' high-lighted the benefits of omega-3s in IBS management, showing that individuals who increased their intake of these fatty acids experienced less abdominal pain and improved bowel regularity. Dr. Mark Pimentel, a leading gastroenterologist emphasize, "Omega-3s have a significant impact on the gut, particularly by reducing low-grade inflammation that is often present in IBS patients. This allows for better gut function and less discomfort."

Leaky Gut and Omega-3's Role in Gut Integrity

Leaky gut syndrome occurs when the intestinal barrier becomes compromised, allowing harmful substances such as toxins and undigested food particles to pass into the bloodstream. This triggers widespread inflammation and is linked to a host of chronic conditions, including autoimmune diseases and metabolic disorders. Omega-3 fatty acids have been shown to support the integrity of the gut lining by reducing inflammation and promoting the production of tight junction proteins that help seal the gut barrier.

Research from the 'Journal of Clinical Gastroenterology' found that omega-3 supplementation in individuals with leaky gut significantly improved gut barrier function, reducing systemic inflammation and alleviating symptoms. Dr. Alessio Fasano, an expert in gut permeability states, "Omega-3s play a crucial role in maintaining the gut lining's integrity. By reducing inflammation and supporting barrier function, they help prevent the progression of leaky gut and its associated health complications."

The Future of Digestive Health

Omega-3 fatty acids are emerging as a vital component in the prevention and treatment of digestive disorders such as IBS and leaky gut syndrome. Their ability to reduce inflammation, support gut integrity, and modulate the gut microbiome offers a holistic solution for those struggling with chronic digestive issues. By incorporating omega-3s into a broader strategy for digestive health, individuals can experience real, lasting relief from the debilitating symptoms of these conditions.

Dr. Eugene Fine, a nutritional scientist, summarizes the impact of omega-3s on gut health, "Omega-3s offer more than just symptom relief. They provide a mechanism for gut healing, inflammation reduction, and restoration of overall digestive balance—critical factors for long-term health and wellness."

The potential of omega-3s in digestive health continues to grow, offering hope to those looking for a natural, effective way to manage their conditions and restore balance to their gut health. Just like with Sarah, a holistic approach is often the answer to long term health issues, something she never considered (or her other doctor's considered).

nine

pregnancy, children, and omega-3s

WHILE MUCH OF this book has focused on the benefits of omega-3 fatty acids for adult health, especially in the context of chronic inflammation and longevity, it's important to recognize that omega-3s play a critical role throughout the entire lifespan. For young families or those planning to have children, omega-3 intake is particularly vital during pregnancy and early childhood. The development of a child's brain, nervous system, and overall health is profoundly influenced by the mother's nutritional intake, with omega-3s being one of the most essential components.

From supporting brain development in the womb to ensuring healthy cognitive function and growth in early childhood, omega-3s—particularly DHA (docosahexaenoic acid)—are a cornerstone of both maternal and child health. In this chapter, we will explore how omega-3s benefit pregnancy and early childhood development, and why prioritizing these fats is crucial for the health and future well-being of both mother and child.

Omega-3 in Pregnancy: Brain and Nervous System Development

During pregnancy, the demand for omega-3 fatty acids—especially DHA—skyrockets, as they are critical for the development of the baby's brain and nervous system. DHA is a primary structural component of the brain and retina, making it essential for cognitive function, visual acuity, and overall neurological development. Studies have consistently shown that adequate omega-3 intake during pregnancy leads to better outcomes for both mother and child, including improved birth weight, reduced risk of preterm birth, and enhanced brain function in the child.

DHA and Fetal Brain Development

The human brain undergoes rapid growth during pregnancy, particularly in the third trimester. DHA is required for this growth, as it makes up a large portion of the brain's gray matter and is crucial for the formation of neurons and synapses. Dr. Sheila Innis, a leading expert in maternal and infant nutrition, explains, "DHA is critical for brain development, particularly during the last trimester of pregnancy when the fetal brain is growing at an exponential rate. Without adequate DHA, the brain and nervous system may not develop optimally."

The importance of DHA for brain development is underscored by several studies showing that children whose mothers had higher levels of omega-3s during pregnancy scored better on cognitive and visual tests during early childhood. A study published in 'The American Journal of Clinical Nutrition' found that children whose mothers supplemented with DHA during pregnancy performed better on problem-solving and language development tests at age 4.

Preventing Preterm Birth and Improving Birth Outcomes

In addition to brain development, omega-3s play a critical role in supporting a healthy pregnancy. Research has shown that adequate omega-3 intake can help reduce the risk of preterm birth, one of the leading causes of neonatal mortality and long-term developmental issues. Omega-3s help support the length of gestation by promoting the production of prostaglandins, which regulate uterine contractions and reduce the likelihood of premature labor.

Dr. Susan Carlson, a leading researcher on omega-3s and pregnancy, states, "Omega-3s, particularly DHA, have been shown to reduce the risk of early preterm birth by as much as 40%. This is a significant finding, as preterm birth is one of the leading causes of infant morbidity and mortality."

Additionally, omega-3s contribute to healthier birth weights and reduce the risk of conditions like preeclampsia, which can be dangerous for both mother and baby. Omega-3s have anti-inflammatory effects that help regulate blood pressure and improve placental function, ensuring that the baby receives adequate oxygen and nutrients during pregnancy.

The Role of Omega-3s in the Nervous System

Beyond the brain, omega-3s are integral to the development of the entire nervous system. DHA supports the formation of the myelin sheath, the protective coating around nerves that ensures proper electrical signal transmission. Without adequate DHA, the development of the nervous system can be compromised, potentially leading to cognitive and motor impairments later in life.

A review published in 'Frontiers in Neuroscience' highlights the role of omega-3s in nervous system health, noting, "DHA is not only critical for the formation of the central nervous system but also for its function. Adequate DHA levels during pregnancy are associated with improved motor skills and cognitive function in the child."

Long-Term Benefits for Child Development

The benefits of omega-3 intake during pregnancy extend well beyond birth. Studies have shown that children whose mothers consumed adequate omega-3s during pregnancy continue to show cognitive and behavioral advantages well into childhood. A study published in 'Pediatrics' found that children who were exposed to higher levels of DHA in the womb had better attention spans, memory, and cognitive flexibility at age 7, compared to those whose mothers had lower DHA levels.

Dr. Joseph Hibbeln, a neuroscientist at the National Institutes of Health explains, "The long-term cognitive benefits of omega-3 intake during pregnancy are well-documented. Children born to mothers with higher DHA levels consistently perform better on cognitive and behavioral tests throughout childhood."

A Critical Nutrient for Mother and Child

Omega-3 fatty acids, particularly DHA, are indispensable during pregnancy for the development of the brain and nervous system, as well as for supporting a healthy pregnancy. The research is clear: ensuring adequate omega-3 intake during pregnancy is one of the most important steps expectant mothers can take to support their child's future cognitive and neurological health.

As more families become aware of the importance of omega-3s, particularly in early life, it is vital to continue spreading the message that these essential fats are not just beneficial but essential for giving children the best possible start in life. For those planning a family or currently expecting, prioritizing omega-3s will lay the foundation for a lifetime of health and well-being for both mother and child.

The recommended concentrations of DHA (docosahexaenoic acid) and EPA (eicosapentaenoic acid) differ for children and adults, largely due to the rapid neurodevelopment that occurs during childhood, especially in the first few years of life. DHA is particularly critical during this period, as it is a key building block for brain and retinal development, whereas EPA plays a more significant role in regulating inflammation and supporting cardiovascular health.

DHA for Children

In children, DHA is emphasized more heavily than EPA due to the rapid development of the brain and nervous system, especially from infancy through early childhood. During the last trimester of pregnancy and the first two years of life, DHA accumulates rapidly in the brain and retina. This high demand for DHA continues during early childhood as cognitive, motor, and visual development peaks. Many health organizations recommend specific DHA intake guidelines to support this critical growth:

Infants: DHA intake is particularly important during infancy. The World Health Organization (WHO) and the Food and Agriculture Organization (FAO) recommend that DHA constitute 0.2-0.36% of total energy intake for infants.

Children aged 1-3 years: The recommended intake of DHA for young children typically ranges from 70-100 mg/day, according to the European Food Safety Authority (EFSA). This supports cognitive function and eye development.

Older children: For children aged 4-8 years, recommendations increase to around 250 mg/day of combined DHA and EPA. This amount supports ongoing brain development, learning, and attention.

Dr. Alex Richardson, a neuroscientist and researcher in child nutrition, states: "DHA is essential for brain growth and function. Without sufficient DHA during early development, children may not reach their full cognitive potential."

DHA and EPA for Adults

For adults, the emphasis shifts slightly to a more balanced intake of DHA and EPA, with EPA playing a larger role due to its anti-inflammatory properties and benefits for heart health. For adults, the recommended daily intake typically ranges from 250-500 mg of combined DHA and EPA. The balance between the two depends on the individual's needs, with EPA taking a more prominent role in managing inflammation and reducing cardiovascular risk, while DHA continues to support brain and eye health.

Adults: The American Heart Association (AHA) recommends consuming at least 500 mg/day of combined DHA and EPA for overall health, with an emphasis on heart disease prevention.

Pregnant and breastfeeding women: DHA is crucial during pregnancy and breastfeeding to support the baby's brain development. Health authorities like the EFSA recommend at least 200 mg/day of DHA in addition to the regular omega-3 intake for pregnant and breastfeeding women.

Why DHA Concentrations Differ

The reason children require higher proportions of DHA compared to adults is due to the unique and rapid brain development that occurs in early life. DHA accounts for a significant portion of the brain's lipid content, particularly in the cerebral cortex and retina, making it indispensable for neurodevelopment. In contrast, adults have largely completed the development of their central nervous system, so their focus shifts toward maintaining brain health, cardiovascular function, and reducing inflammation.

As Dr. Michael Crawford, a pioneer in brain nutrition notes, "DHA is the most important fatty acid for the developing brain. The rapid brain growth during childhood requires substantial amounts of DHA to support cognitive, motor, and visual development."

In summary, while both DHA and EPA are important for overall health, children have a greater need for DHA to support brain and retinal development, whereas adults benefit from a more balanced intake to address broader health needs, including inflammation and cardiovascular protection.

Holistic Nutritional Recommendations for DHA and EPA

Many alternative doctors, functional medicine practitioners, and naturopaths find the typical recommended daily dosages for omega-3 fatty acids—both DHA and EPA—to be far too low, especially for those looking to optimize health and address specific concerns like inflammation, brain development, and chronic disease prevention. Here's a breakdown of what these experts typically recommend for various groups, with a focus on higher therapeutic doses of DHA and EPA.

DHA for Children: Recommendations That Differ Than FDA and Health Canada Recommendations

Functional medicine practitioners tend to recommend higher amounts of DHA for children than conventional guidelines, particularly because of its role in supporting rapid brain and nervous system development.

Infants: While conventional recommendations suggest DHA intake of 70-100 mg/day, alternative doctors often recommend between 150-300 mg/day of DHA for infants, particularly for those who are breastfed or have developmental concerns.

Children aged 1-3 years: For young children, alternative doctors may recommend a DHA intake of 200-400 mg/day. This is to optimize cognitive development, visual acuity, and support for early neurological growth, which is often more significant than conventional guidance accounts for.

Older children (4-8 years): Functional medicine experts often suggest combined DHA and EPA dosages of 500-800 mg/day, with an emphasis on DHA for children, to support learning, attention, and behavioral regulation. Many practitioners recommend a DHA to EPA ratio favoring DHA, around 2:1.

Dr. David Perlmutter, a neurologist and expert in brain health states, "The conventional omega-3 recommendations for children are generally too low. Higher levels of DHA, especially in the first few years of life, are critical for optimal brain development and cognitive performance."

DHA and EPA for Adults: Holistic Nutrition Advice

Adults: Instead of the typical 500 mg/day of combined DHA and EPA recommended by conventional guidelines, many naturopaths suggest a range of 1,000-3,000 mg/day, with some practitioners pushing as high as 4,000-5,000 mg/day for individuals with inflammatory conditions or cardiovascular concerns. A balance of around 60% EPA to 40% DHA is common for adult health needs.

Dr. Mark Hyman, a well-known figure in functional medicine, advocates for higher omega-3 intake explaining, "For most adults, especially those with chronic inflammation or cognitive decline, the standard recommendations are inadequate. I routinely recommend 2,000-3,000 mg of combined DHA and EPA per day to optimize brain function and reduce inflammation."

Pregnant and Breastfeeding Women

For pregnant and breastfeeding women, functional medicine experts generally emphasize a higher DHA intake to support fetal brain development and maternal health, far beyond conventional recommendations.

Pregnant and breastfeeding women: Alternative doctors often recommend at least 500-700 mg/day of DHA, in addition to 500-1,000 mg/day of EPA, resulting in a total omega-3 intake of around 1,500-2,000 mg/day. This supports both the developing baby's brain and the mother's mental and physical health.

Dr. Aviva Romm, a specialist in women's health suggests, "During pregnancy, I recommend women take 500 mg to 1,000 mg of DHA per day to support their baby's brain development, along with EPA for its anti-inflammatory effects."

Why Higher Dosages?

Neurodevelopment: The growing brain of a child is especially dependent on high concentrations of DHA, as it forms the structure of brain cells and is crucial for synaptic development. Conventional guidelines often underestimate the true need for DHA during these critical stages of growth.

Chronic Inflammation: Many functional medicine doctors prescribe higher omega-3 doses to combat systemic inflammation, which is implicated in diseases like arthritis, heart disease, and autoimmune conditions. Dr. Joseph Mercola, a prominent alternative medicine advocate, often recommends omega-3 supplementation at 3,000-4,000 mg/day for those with inflammatory disorders.

Functional medicine and naturopathic practitioners advocate for much higher DHA and EPA intakes compared to conventional guidelines, particularly for children's neurodevelopment, pregnancy, and managing chronic inflammatory conditions. They often prescribe anywhere from 2-5 times the conventional recommendations, arguing that these higher doses better reflect the body's true needs in today's modern health landscape.

Dr. Sarah Ballantyne, a medical researcher underscores this point, "The therapeutic benefits of omega-3s are dose-dependent. Most people would benefit from significantly higher intakes than what is typically recommended."

These higher dosages, used in consultation with healthcare professionals, can offer more profound health benefits for both children and adults looking to optimize cognitive and cardiovascular health, reduce inflammation, and support long-term well-being.

Essential Nutrients for Growing Kids: The Role of Omega-3

As children grow, their bodies require a wide array of essential nutrients to support rapid physical and cognitive development. While macronutrients like protein and carbohydrates get plenty of attention, omega-3 fatty acids are among the most critical yet often overlooked nutrients in a child's diet. These fatty acids, particularly DHA (docosahexaenoic acid) and EPA (eicosapentaenoic acid), are essential for brain development, immune function, and overall cellular health.

Cognitive and Behavioral Development

One of the most important roles omega-3s play in growing children is in brain development and cognitive function. The brain is composed of nearly 60% fat, and DHA makes up a significant portion of that. DHA is required for the formation of the brain's structure, including neurons and synaptic connections, which are critical for learning, memory, and emotional regulation.

Dr. David Perlmutter, a neurologist highlights, "Children with higher levels of DHA have been shown to perform better in areas such as reading, learning, and behavior. This is not just during early development but throughout childhood as well."

Numerous studies have shown that children with adequate omega-3 levels tend to have improved attention, focus, and cognitive flexibility. For example, a study published in 'The American Journal of Clinical Nutrition' demonstrated that omega-3 supplementation in school-aged children improved attention spans and reduced impulsivity—an effect that was particularly beneficial for children with ADHD (Attention Deficit Hyperactivity Disorder).

Immune Function and Inflammation Control

Growing kids are exposed to a variety of pathogens as their immune systems develop, and omega-3s play an important role in modulating immune responses and controlling inflammation. Omega-3 fatty acids help regulate the production of inflammatory molecules, such as cytokines, and maintain a healthy immune balance. Children who have a diet rich in omega-3s tend to have better immune function and may be less prone to chronic inflammatory conditions like asthma and eczema.

A review published in 'Nutrients' highlighted the role of omega-3s in childhood immune health, stating: "Children who consume adequate levels of omega-3 fatty acids have been shown to have stronger immune responses and lower rates of inflammatory conditions, including asthma and allergies."

Bone and Joint Health

As children grow, their skeletal systems are constantly developing, and omega-3s can aid in maintaining joint flexibility and reducing the risk of inflammation in growing bones. Omega-3 fatty acids support the formation of healthy cartilage and help protect the joints from wear and tear, which is particularly important for children who are active in sports or other physical activities.

Dr. Susan Blum, an expert in functional medicine, emphasizes: "Omega-3s help reduce inflammation in growing joints, protecting children who are active from injury and supporting overall bone health."

Supporting Vision and Eye Health

Omega-3s, particularly DHA, are also crucial for the development of a child's visual system. DHA is a key structural component of the retina, the part of the eye responsible for translating light into signals that the brain interprets as vision. Adequate levels of DHA are necessary for maintaining sharp visual acuity and overall eye health as children grow.

A study from 'Investigative Ophthalmology & Visual Science' found that children with higher DHA levels had better vision development and a lower risk of visual impairments compared to those with low DHA intake.

Emotional and Behavioral Stability

In addition to cognitive development, omega-3s play a role in emotional and behavioral health. DHA and EPA have been shown to influence mood regulation, with studies indicating that omega-3 deficiencies in children may be linked to mood swings, anxiety, and even depressive symptoms.

A study published in 'European Child & Adolescent Psychiatry' found that children with higher omega-3 levels exhibited fewer emotional and behavioral issues, including symptoms of anxiety and depression. Dr. Joseph Hibbeln, a leader in the study of omega-3s and mental health, notes: "Omega-3s help stabilize mood and promote emotional resilience, making them especially important for children as they navigate the challenges of growing up."

Omega-3s for Lifelong Health

Omega-3s are more than just another nutrient in a child's diet; they are foundational to many aspects of development, from brain function and emotional health to immune system strength and physical growth. Ensuring that children receive enough DHA and EPA during their formative years can set them on a path toward lifelong health, giving them the tools they need to succeed both mentally and physically.

As children grow and develop, omega-3s should be seen as essential nutrients for building strong, healthy bodies and minds.

ADHD and Behavioral Health: The Omega-3 Connection

Research on the role of omega-3 fatty acids, particularly EPA (eicosapentaenoic acid) and DHA (docosahexaenoic acid), in addressing ADHD symptoms has gained significant attention over the last decade. ADHD is a neurodevelopmental disorder characterized by inattention, hyperactivity, and impulsivity, and many children with ADHD have been found to have lower levels of omega-3s in their blood compared to their peers. This deficiency suggests that boosting omega-3 intake may help improve behavioral health and cognitive function in children with ADHD.

How Omega-3s Impact ADHD Symptoms

Several studies have shown that omega-3 supplementation can reduce symptoms of ADHD, such as hyperactivity, impulsivity, and inattentiveness. A study from the UK and Taiwan involving 92 children with ADHD revealed that omega-3 supplementation, particularly EPA, improved the children's ability to focus and maintain attention. However, this benefit was most pronounced in children who had low baseline levels of EPA, highlighting the importance of individualized treatment.

Dr. Carmine Pariante from King's College London, co-lead on the study notes, "For children with omega-3 deficiency, fish oil supplements could be a preferable option to standard stimulant treatments, especially for those not responding well to conventional medication." This approach to "personalized psychiatry" may open new avenues for ADHD management, as omega-3s can provide a natural, non-pharmacological alternative for families seeking complementary treatments.

EPA vs. DHA: What Works Best?

When it comes to the therapeutic effects of omega-3s for ADHD, the balance between EPA and DHA has been a point of focus. While both are beneficial, studies suggest that EPA may play a more direct role in reducing ADHD symptoms, particularly hyperactivity and inattention. For example, a meta-analysis reviewed by 'Psychology Today' found that ADHD patients tend to have lower concentrations of both EPA and DHA in their plasma, but EPA supplementation showed more consistent benefits in improving behavioral symptoms.

In another study published in 'CHADD', researchers found that children who received EPA-rich fish oil experienced significant improvements in ADHD-related behavior compared to those who received DHA alone. This evidence has led to a growing belief that a higher EPA-to-DHA ratio may be most effective for ADHD treatment, particularly for managing hyperactivity and impulsive behavior.

Omega-3s and Cognitive Function in ADHD

Beyond behavioral improvements, omega-3s have also shown promise in supporting cognitive function in children with ADHD. Cognitive flexibility, attention span, and working memory—all areas where children with ADHD often struggle—have been shown to improve with increased omega-3 intake. Studies have demonstrated that children with ADHD who supplemented with omega-3s showed better performance on cognitive tests, such as problem-solving and language tasks.

Dr. James Lake, a psychiatrist specializing in alternative treatments for mental health disorders, explains that omega-3s help improve brain function by affecting neuronal membrane fluidity and reducing inflammation in the brain. He states, "The therapeutic potential of omega-3s lies in their ability to modulate brain function, enhancing cognition and emotional regulation in children with ADHD."

Long-Term Benefits and Recommendations

While omega-3s may not replace conventional ADHD medications for every child, they offer a natural complement to stimulant treatments, especially in children with low omega-3 levels or in cases where medications alone are insufficient. Functional medicine practitioners often recommend omega-3 supplements for ADHD due to their minimal side effects and broad health benefits, including improved mood regulation and reduced inflammation.

A common recommendation is to include at least 1,000-2,000 mg/day of combined EPA and DHA for children with ADHD, with an emphasis on a higher ratio of EPA to DHA, as this has been shown to provide the most consistent results in reducing ADHD symptoms.

In conclusion, omega-3 fatty acids, particularly EPA, hold great potential for reducing ADHD symptoms and improving behavioral health. By incorporating omega-3s into a broader treatment plan, children with ADHD may experience enhanced focus, reduced hyperactivity, and better emotional regulation, offering families a hopeful and holistic approach to managing the disorder.

How to Ensure Optimal Omega-3s During Pregnancy and Early Childhood

Ensuring that both mother and child receive adequate omega-3 fatty acids—especially DHA and EPA—is one of the most important steps to support brain development, immune function, and overall health during pregnancy and early childhood. While many people understand the benefits of omega-3s, it can still be challenging to achieve optimal intake, particularly in an era of processed foods and modern dietary challenges. Here are strategies to ensure optimal omega-3 levels during these critical stages of development.

1. Prioritize High-Quality Omega-3 Sources During Pregnancy

During pregnancy, a mother's nutritional needs change dramatically, and DHA is at the top of the list of essential nutrients for fetal brain development. DHA accumulates rapidly in the fetal brain during the last trimester, making it crucial for neurological development, visual acuity, and cognitive function. Ensuring that pregnant women consume enough omega-3s is not only critical for the child's future health but also for the mother's well-being, as omega-3s can reduce the risk of postpartum depression.

Dr. Joseph Hibbeln, a researcher at the National Institutes of Health notes, "DHA intake during pregnancy is directly related to the future cognitive development of the child. Pregnant women should be consuming 300-500 mg/day of DHA to meet the demands of their growing baby's brain."

Many prenatal vitamins now include DHA, but it's also important to focus on whole food sources like fatty fish (salmon, mackerel, sardines) that provide a bioavailable form of omega-3s. However, due to concerns about mercury in fish, many experts recommend high-quality, purified fish oil supplements as an additional source.

2. Breastfeeding and Omega-3s: A Continued Need

For breastfeeding mothers, DHA continues to be a critical nutrient as it's passed through breast milk and supports the infant's ongoing brain development. The DHA content in breast milk is directly related to the mother's diet, making omega-3 supplementation or consumption of omega-3-rich foods vital for nursing mothers.

Dr. Susan Carlson, a professor of nutrition, states: "The DHA found in breast milk is the primary source of this nutrient for infants, and higher DHA levels in the mother's diet correlate with better cognitive outcomes in children." Breastfeeding mothers should aim for 200-300 mg of DHA per day to ensure their infants receive the optimal amount through breast milk.

3. Omega-3 Supplementation for Infants and Toddlers

For families who may not breastfeed or those transitioning to solid foods, ensuring that children get enough DHA and EPA through their early years remains critical. While infant formulas are now fortified with DHA, pediatricians often recommend omega-3 supplements for toddlers and young children, especially if their diet lacks fatty fish or plant-based sources of ALA (alpha-linolenic acid), which can convert to DHA and EPA in small amounts.

Dr. William Sears, a pediatrician and author emphasizes, "Ensuring adequate omega-3 intake in the early years is essential for brain growth, behavior, and overall health. Parents should look for high-quality omega-3 supplements specifically designed for young children."

Omega-3 supplements in liquid form or chewable gels can be an easy solution for parents who want to ensure their children get enough of this essential nutrient.

4. Balancing Omega-6 and Omega-3 Ratios

While increasing omega-3 intake is crucial, many experts stress the importance of balancing omega-3s with omega-6 fatty acids, which are abundant in modern diets due to processed foods and vegetable oils. As we've already discussed, high intake of omega-6s can compete with omega-3s in the body, reducing their effectiveness.

Dr. Artemis Simopoulos, an expert in essential fatty acid research notes, "The ideal omega-6 to omega-3 ratio should be around 2:1 or 3:1, but in most Western diets, it's closer to 16:1. This imbalance reduces the anti-inflammatory and neuroprotective benefits of omega-3s." Families should aim to reduce sources of omega-6s, such as ultra processed foods and vegetable oils, while boosting omega-3 intake through fish, supplements, and plant-based sources like flaxseeds and walnuts.

5. Omega-3s for Neurodevelopment and Immunity

Omega-3s are not only essential for brain development but also for building a strong immune system. During pregnancy and early childhood, omega-3s support the development of a balanced immune response, reducing the risk of allergies, eczema, and asthma.

Dr. Philip Calder, an immunology expert explains, "Omega-3 fatty acids play a critical role in regulating the immune system, particularly in early life. Children who receive adequate omega-3s during pregnancy and infancy are less likely to develop inflammatory conditions later on."

By ensuring that children have optimal omega-3 levels, parents can support both cognitive and immune development, setting a strong foundation for lifelong health.

A Lifelong Investment in Health

Omega-3 fatty acids, particularly DHA and EPA, are indispensable during pregnancy and early childhood. From supporting brain development and cognitive function to ensuring a balanced immune system, omega-3s lay the foundation for a healthy future. By prioritizing omega-3-rich foods, supplements, and balancing the overall diet, families can help children reach their full developmental potential.

As Dr. Sheila Innis, a renowned expert in maternal and child nutrition, puts it: "Ensuring optimal omega-3 intake during these critical stages is one of the most important things parents can do to support their child's health and development."

ten

omega-6 – the overlooked problem

WHEN SARAH first began her health journey, much of her focus was on improving her own well-being—particularly her posture and digestive issues. Over time, however, she developed a deeper understanding of how the modern food industry operates and how it affects not just her health, but the health of her children as well. As Sarah learned more about omega-3s and omega-6s, she became aware of a disturbing reality: food producers have shifted to using low-quality, highly processed food substitutes that are often rich in omega-6 fatty acids. These substitutes, like vegetable oils and processed snacks, are subsidized by the government to keep costs down but come with an enormous health cost.

Sarah realized that the cheap convenience of these products was eroding her family's health from the inside out. Armed with this new knowledge, Sarah started to make better choices—not only for herself but for her children too. Her understanding of the omega-3 to omega-6 balance was now helping her navigate the overwhelming world of modern food marketing, and her children were benefiting from a healthier, more thoughtful diet. What once seemed like small, insignificant changes were now making a tangible difference in her family's energy, focus, and overall well-being.

Why Omega-6 Isn't the Enemy: Understanding Its Role

While much of the attention around omega-3 and omega-6 fatty acids paints omega-6 as the "bad guy," the reality is that omega-6 isn't inherently harmful. In fact, omega-6 fatty acids, like linoleic acid, are essential for many bodily functions, including brain development, skin health, and regulating metabolism. The real problem isn't omega-6 itself—it's the disproportionate amount we consume today compared to omega-3s.

The Role of Omega-6 in the Body

Omega-6 is part of the essential fatty acids family, meaning our bodies cannot produce it, and we must obtain it through our diet. Omega-6 plays an important role in inflammation regulation, as it helps produce signaling molecules called prostaglandins. In moderation, these molecules are necessary for the body's immune response, particularly in healing wounds and fighting infections. Dr. Artemis Simopoulos emphasizes, "Omega-6 fatty acids are essential for health, but when consumed in excess, they can promote chronic inflammation, which leads to diseases such as heart disease, diabetes, and obesity."

The issue arises from the imbalance between omega-6 and omega-3 fatty acids in the average modern diet. Historically, humans consumed omega-6 and omega-3 in a ratio of about 1:1. Today, with the advent of processed foods and cheap vegetable oils, the typical Western diet has a ratio closer to 16:1 or even 20:1. This imbalance leads to chronic inflammation, which is linked to many modern diseases.

Why the Government and Food Industry Aren't Fixing This

I briefly touched on this earlier in the book, but one of the most troubling aspects of the omega-6 problem is how deeply embedded it is in the modern food system. The production of vegetable oils like corn, soybean, and sunflower oil—rich in omega-6—is heavily subsidized by governments. These oils are inexpensive to produce, have a long shelf life, and are found in countless ultra processed foods, from salad dressings to snack chips. This system benefits large food companies that prioritize profit over health, leaving consumers to deal with the consequences.

Dr. Mark Hyman comments, "The food industry, supported by government subsidies, is pumping our diets full of unhealthy omega-6s, contributing to a chronic imbalance that fuels inflammation and disease. We cannot rely on the government or food manufacturers to protect our health—we must take responsibility for what we eat."

The food lobby plays a significant role in shaping food policies and guidelines, often favoring these cheap, omega-6-heavy ingredients. As a result, many processed foods marketed as "healthy" are still loaded with harmful omega-6 oils. This means that consumers need to be informed and proactive, making conscious decisions about the types of fats they consume.

Taking Control of Our Health

While omega-6 fatty acids are necessary, the key is to reduce their intake and restore balance by increasing omega-3 consumption. Dr. Andrew Weil, a pioneer in integrative medicine advises, "Reducing the intake of processed foods and vegetable oils while boosting omega-3-rich foods like wild-caught fish, flaxseeds, and chia seeds is the best way to restore a healthy balance and reduce inflammation."

One important step is reading food labels carefully and avoiding products that list vegetable oils high in omega-6, such as soybean, corn, and sunflower oils. Instead, opt for healthier fats like olive oil, avocado oil, and fats from omega-3-rich sources like fatty fish. Dr. Joseph Mercola adds, "Avoiding omega-6-rich processed foods and shifting to whole, nutrient-dense foods is crucial for bringing the omega-3 and omega-6 ratio back into balance and protecting our health."

It's Up to Us

In today's food environment, where profit often outweighs public health, it's clear that we cannot rely on external forces to safeguard our well-being. Sarah's newfound understanding of omega-6 and omega-3 balance is a perfect example of how knowledge can empower individuals to take control of their health. By being mindful of the fats we consume and striving to reduce our intake of omega-6-rich processed foods, we can protect our bodies from chronic inflammation and ensure a healthier future for ourselves and our families. The change begins with us, and it's within our power to make a difference.

How Too Much Omega-6 Disrupts Health

While omega-6 fatty acids are essential for normal bodily function, the overconsumption of these fats—especially in the form of processed vegetable oils—has become a major health concern. In the modern diet, the balance between omega-6 and omega-3 fatty acids has shifted dramatically, leading to an imbalance that can fuel chronic inflammation, increase the risk of heart disease, and contribute to other long-term health issues. Understanding how excess omega-6 disrupts health is crucial for making informed dietary choices.

1. Chronic Inflammation

One of the primary ways excess omega-6 fatty acids affect health is by promoting chronic inflammation. Omega-6 fats, particularly linoleic acid, are precursors to inflammatory molecules called eicosanoids. While these molecules are essential for the immune response and healing processes, too much omega-6 leads to an overproduction of pro-inflammatory eicosanoids. This can result in low-grade, chronic inflammation, which is linked to a wide array of diseases.

Dr. Artemis Simopoulos, explains: "The typical Western diet contains far too much omega-6 and not enough omega-3. This imbalance promotes inflammation, which is a major factor in many chronic diseases such as heart disease, cancer, and autoimmune conditions." Research has shown that individuals with a high intake of omega-6 relative to omega-3s have higher levels of inflammatory markers in their blood, putting them at greater risk of developing inflammatory conditions.

2. Increased Risk of Cardiovascular Disease

Omega-6 fatty acids, when consumed in excess, can also contribute to cardiovascular disease. The inflammatory nature of omega-6 fats can lead to the development of plaque in the arteries, increasing the risk of atherosclerosis, heart attacks, and strokes. While omega-6 fats can lower LDL ("bad") cholesterol, their pro-inflammatory effects may outweigh these benefits, particularly in the context of an omega-6/omega-3 imbalance.

Dr. William Harris, a renowned expert in cardiovascular health points out, "While omega-6 fatty acids have been shown to lower cholesterol, the real issue lies in their inflammatory potential. When consumed in excess, omega-6 fats can contribute to the very heart diseases we are trying to prevent." Harris emphasizes the importance of balancing omega-6 with omega-3 to reduce inflammation and protect heart health.

3. Impairment of Mental Health and Cognitive Function

Excessive omega-6 intake, particularly when it overwhelms omega-3 levels, has been linked to mental health issues, including depression, anxiety, and cognitive decline. Omega-6 fats, through their pro-inflammatory eicosanoids, can negatively impact brain function by increasing inflammation in the brain. This is concerning because chronic brain inflammation has been linked to neurodegenerative diseases such as Alzheimer's.

Dr. Joseph Hibbeln from the National Institutes of Health, who has extensively studied the relationship between omega fatty acids and mental health, states, "There is compelling evidence that diets high in omega-6, particularly in relation to omega-3 intake, contribute to higher rates of depression and cognitive dysfunction. Reducing omega-6 and increasing omega-3 can help protect mental health." Hibbeln's research suggests that the balance of omega-3 to omega-6 fats is crucial for maintaining optimal brain function and emotional stability.

4. Obesity and Metabolic Disorders

Omega-6 fatty acids have also been implicated in the rise of obesity and metabolic disorders. Excess omega-6 intake, particularly in the form of processed vegetable oils, can disrupt insulin sensitivity and promote fat storage. The chronic low-grade inflammation caused by omega-6 fats may impair the body's ability to regulate glucose, contributing to insulin resistance, a precursor to type 2 diabetes.

A study published in 'The Journal of Lipid Research' found that high levels of omega-6 fatty acids, especially linoleic acid, were associated with increased fat storage and impaired metabolic function. Dr. Dariush Mozaffarian, a cardiovascular epidemiologist notes, "Omega-6s are not inherently harmful, but when consumed in excess, particularly in an imbalanced diet, they can contribute to metabolic dysfunction and increased fat deposition."

5. Contribution to Autoimmune Diseases

Autoimmune diseases, such as rheumatoid arthritis, lupus, and multiple sclerosis, are also closely tied to chronic inflammation. Given that omega-6 fatty acids promote inflammation, diets high in omega-6 can exacerbate the symptoms of autoimmune diseases. The inflammatory compounds produced by omega-6s can stimulate an overactive immune response, where the body begins attacking its own tissues.

Functional medicine expert Dr. Mark Hyman comments, "Many patients with autoimmune conditions have found that reducing omega-6 intake, particularly from processed foods and vegetable oils, helps reduce symptoms by lowering inflammation in the body." This underscores the importance of not only increasing omega-3 intake but also minimizing omega-6 consumption to manage inflammation and improve immune function.

Finding Balance for Better Health

The issue with omega-6 isn't that it's inherently harmful—it's that the modern diet provides an overwhelming excess, leading to a cascade of health problems. The key to maintaining health is not to eliminate omega-6 fatty acids but to restore the balance between omega-6 and omega-3. By reducing the intake of processed foods, vegetable oils, and increasing omega-3-rich foods like fatty fish and flaxseeds, we can help protect our bodies from chronic inflammation, heart disease, mental health issues, and autoimmune conditions.

As Dr. Andrew Weil concludes, "Achieving the right balance between omega-3 and omega-6 fatty acids is one of the most important steps we can take for our health. It requires awareness and intentional choices, but the impact on overall well-being is profound."

This chapter serves as a reminder that while omega-6 is essential, too

much of a good thing can disrupt our health. It's up to each of us to make informed choices and find the balance that supports long-term wellness.

Strategies to Reduce Omega-6 in Your Diet

Reducing your intake of omega-6 fatty acids is an essential step toward restoring a healthier balance between omega-6 and omega-3 fats in the diet. Omega-6 fats are present in almost all modern ultra processed foods, making them nearly unavoidable unless intentional dietary changes are made. The key to success is recognizing the common sources of omega-6 and making informed substitutions that support overall health.

1. Avoid Processed and Packaged Foods

One of the simplest ways to reduce omega-6 intake is to limit processed and packaged foods, which are often laden with omega-6-rich oils like soybean, corn, and sunflower oil. These oils are used because they are inexpensive, have a long shelf life, and are highly processed.

Dr. Mark Hyman notes: "The modern Western diet is filled with hidden omega-6 fats, especially in processed snacks, salad dressings, and fast food. By eliminating or reducing these foods, you can significantly lower your omega-6 intake."

2. Replace Vegetable Oils with Healthier Alternatives

Vegetable oils high in omega-6, such as soybean, corn, safflower, and sunflower oils, are commonly used in cooking and food preparation. Replacing these with healthier alternatives can drastically shift your omega-6 intake. Opt for oils like extra-virgin olive oil, avocado oil, and coconut oil, which have healthier fatty acid profiles.

Dr. Artemis Simopoulos explains: "One of the most effective ways to reduce omega-6 intake is to replace omega-6-rich oils with healthier oils like olive oil, which contains monounsaturated fats and a small amount of omega-3."

3. Choose Whole, Unprocessed Foods

Focusing on whole, unprocessed foods like fresh vegetables, fruits, whole grains, nuts, and seeds can help minimize omega-6 intake. Most whole foods contain relatively low levels of omega-6 and provide essential nutrients that support overall health. Wild-caught fish, grass-fed meat, and pasture-raised eggs are particularly beneficial sources of omega-3 that can help rebalance the ratio of omega-6 to omega-3.

Dr. Joseph Mercola emphasizes: "By prioritizing whole, unprocessed foods, you avoid the excessive omega-6 found in processed oils and packaged products. A diet based on real food naturally brings your omega-6 intake down to healthier levels."

4. Be Mindful of Restaurant Meals

Many restaurants, particularly fast food and chain establishments, use oils high in omega-6 to cook and prepare their dishes. To reduce omega-6 intake when dining out, opt for grilled or steamed dishes, avoid fried foods, and ask if your meal can be cooked with healthier oils like olive oil or avocado oil.

Dr. Andrew Weil suggests, "When eating out, be cautious of foods prepared with cheap vegetable oils. Asking for your food to be grilled or roasted without added oils can help minimize your intake of omega-6."

Practical Tips: How to Shift the Ratio for Optimal Health

Shifting the balance between omega-6 and omega-3 fatty acids toward a healthier ratio requires mindful eating and thoughtful food choices. While reducing omega-6 intake is one part of the equation, increasing your omega-3 intake is just as important to achieve the right balance for optimal health.

1. Prioritize Omega-3-Rich Foods

One of the best ways to improve the omega-6 to omega-3 ratio is to increase your intake of foods rich in omega-3s, such as fatty fish, flaxseeds, chia seeds, walnuts, and grass-fed animal products. Fatty fish like salmon, mackerel, and sardines are particularly high in EPA and DHA, the most bioavailable forms of omega-3.

Dr. William Harris emphasizes: "The best way to improve your omega-3 levels is to eat more fatty fish. Even just two servings a week of wild-caught fish can significantly boost your omega-3 intake and help shift the balance."

2. Consider Omega-3 Supplements

For individuals who find it difficult to get enough omega-3 from food alone, high-quality fish oil or algae-based supplements are a convenient and effective way to increase omega-3 intake. Look for supplements that provide a balance of EPA and DHA, as these forms are the most effective for reducing inflammation and supporting brain and heart health.

Dr. Michael Lewis recommends: "For those who don't eat fish regularly, omega-3 supplements are an excellent way to ensure you're getting enough of these critical fatty acids. Just make sure you choose a supplement with a high EPA and DHA content for the best results."

3. Limit Omega-6-Rich Snacks

Many snacks, including chips, crackers, and baked goods, are high in omega-6 fats due to the use of vegetable oils. Opt for healthier snack options that are low in omega-6, such as raw nuts, seeds, or whole fruits. These alternatives not only reduce omega-6 intake but also provide other essential nutrients.

Dr. Sarah Ballantyne, a medical researcher and author suggests, "Swap out processed snacks for whole foods like nuts and seeds, which provide healthy fats and protein without the omega-6 overload."

4. Cook at Home More Often

One of the most effective strategies to control your omega-6 and omega-3 intake is to cook at home, where you can choose the types of oils and ingredients used in your meals. This gives you complete control over the quality of your fats and allows you to prioritize healthier options.

Dr. Mark Hyman notes, "Cooking at home is one of the most powerful ways to improve your omega-6 to omega-3 ratio. You can avoid harmful oils and create balanced meals using omega-3-rich ingredients."

5. Focus on Balance, Not Elimination

As I've mentioned earlier, the goal is not to eliminate omega-6 entirely, as it plays a necessary role in the body, but to achieve a healthier balance. Strive to reduce omega-6 intake while boosting omega-3s, aiming for a ratio closer to 1:1 or 2:1. This balance helps reduce inflammation, improve heart health, and support overall wellness.

Dr. Artemis Simopoulos sums it up, "Omega-6 is not the enemy—

it's the imbalance that's harmful. By increasing omega-3 intake and reducing excess omega-6, you can restore your body's natural equilibrium and protect your health."

By following these strategies and practical tips, you can shift your omega-6 to omega-3 ratio to a healthier balance, reducing inflammation and promoting long-term well-being for you and your family. The power to optimize your health lies in your food choices, and with mindfulness and planning, you can achieve the balance necessary for vibrant health.

the practical omega solution – fixing your fats

IN THIS CHAPTER, we bring everything together to provide practical steps to help you fix your fats and achieve a healthier balance between omega-3 and omega-6 fatty acids. Yes, you will see some common themes that have already been presented in more detail, but I wanted to recap the concepts in a step by step summary. By following these guidelines, you can not only reduce inflammation and improve your overall health, but also make smarter choices when it comes to fat consumption.

How to Measure Your Omega-3 to Omega-6 Ratio

Understanding your omega-3 to omega-6 ratio is one of the first steps toward optimizing your fat intake. The ideal ratio is around 1:1 to 2:1 (omega-6 to omega-3), but the average Western diet often skews this ratio to 16:1 or worse. This imbalance contributes to chronic inflammation and many modern diseases.

There are now simple ways to measure this ratio, such as at-home omega-3 test kits that analyze the fatty acid profile in your blood. These tests provide a snapshot of the balance between omega-3s and omega-6s and help you understand where you need to adjust your intake. Dr. William Harris explains, "By measuring your omega-3 levels, you can identify whether your diet is supporting or harming your health. It's important to know where you stand so you can make the necessary adjustments."

A 2016 study published in the 'Journal of Nutritional Biochemistry' found that individuals with a better omega-6 to omega-3 ratio had significantly lower levels of inflammation and reduced risk of chronic diseases such as heart disease and metabolic disorders. This research supports the value of tracking and optimizing this ratio.

The Best Sources of Omega-3: From Food to Supplements

The key to fixing your omega-3 to omega-6 ratio is to prioritize foods rich in omega-3s while reducing omega-6 intake from processed foods and vegetable oils. Here are the best sources of omega-3s:

Fatty Fish: Wild-caught salmon, mackerel, sardines, and anchovies are the richest natural sources of EPA and DHA, the most bioavailable forms of omega-3. Dr. Andrew Weil states, "Fatty fish should be a regular part of your diet if you want to optimize your omega-3 levels." Aim for at least two servings of fatty fish per week.

Flaxseeds and Chia Seeds: For plant-based omega-3s, flaxseeds and chia seeds provide ALA (alpha-linolenic acid), which can be partially converted to EPA and DHA. While the conversion rate is low, these foods are still valuable sources of omega-3. Dr. Michael Greger notes, "Flaxseeds are an excellent addition to any diet and can help boost omega-3 levels for those who don't consume fish."

Algal Oil: For vegans or those allergic to fish, algal oil supplements provide a direct source of DHA. A study published in 'The Journal of Nutrition' found that algal oil is just as effective as fish oil in raising DHA levels in the body.

Grass-Fed Meat and Pasture-Raised Eggs: Grass-fed meats and pasture-raised eggs contain higher levels of omega-3s compared to their grain-fed counterparts. Dr. Joseph Mercola recommends choosing these sources as part of a balanced diet to support healthy fat intake.

Cooking with Healthy Fats: A Practical Guide to Everyday Eating

Choosing the right fats for cooking is an essential part of optimizing your omega-3 to omega-6 ratio. Many oils used in cooking are high in omega-6, so it's important to replace them with healthier options.

Use Olive Oil: Extra-virgin olive oil is rich in monounsaturated fats and low in omega-6, making it an excellent choice for everyday cooking. Dr. Artemis Simopoulos notes, "Olive oil is not only heart-healthy but also a key component in reducing omega-6 intake. It's a great replacement for vegetable oils in most dishes."

Cook with Avocado Oil: Avocado oil has a high smoke point, making it ideal for cooking at higher temperatures. It is low in omega-6 and rich in heart-healthy monounsaturated fats.

Avoid Soybean and Corn Oils: These oils are high in omega-6 and are commonly found in processed foods and snacks. Dr. Mark Hyman advises, "Stay away from oils like soybean and corn oil. They are contributing to the imbalance of fats in your diet and are highly inflammatory."

Coconut Oil for High-Heat Cooking: Coconut oil is a saturated fat with a high smoke point, making it ideal for high-temperature cooking. Although it doesn't provide omega-3s, it is a stable, healthy fat for cooking that won't oxidize like vegetable oils.

Supplementing Smartly: When and How to Add Omega-3s to Your Diet

For many people, even a diet rich in omega-3 foods may not provide enough DHA and EPA to optimize their health. This is where supplements come in. Choosing the right supplement and using it correctly can make all the difference in achieving optimal omega-3 levels.

Fish Oil Supplements: These are the most common and effective omega-3 supplements, rich in both EPA and DHA. Look for high-quality fish oils that are molecularly distilled to remove impurities like mercury and PCBs. Dr. William Harris emphasizes, "Fish oil supplements are an excellent way to ensure you're getting enough omega-3s, especially if you're not eating fish regularly."

Krill Oil: Krill oil is another option, with the added benefit of containing antioxidants like astaxanthin. A study published in 'Lipids in Health and Disease' showed that krill oil may be more bioavailable than fish oil due to its phospholipid structure, which allows for better absorption in the body.

Algal Oil for Vegetarians and Vegans: Algal oil provides DHA directly from algae, making it an excellent option for plant-based diets. Research has shown that algal oil can effectively raise omega-3 levels and is a sustainable alternative to fish oil.

Dr. Michael Lewis advises, "When choosing a supplement, ensure it provides a high concentration of EPA and DHA. Most people need 1,000-2,000 mg per day for optimal health, but always consult your healthcare provider before starting."

Avoiding Common Pitfalls: Mistakes People Make with Fats

Despite the benefits of omega-3 supplementation, many people make mistakes when trying to improve their fat intake. Here are some common pitfalls and how to avoid them:

Relying Too Much on Plant-Based Omega-3s: While flaxseeds and chia seeds are great sources of ALA, the body's conversion rate of ALA to EPA and DHA is very low—often less than 10%. Dr. Sarah Ballantyne warns, "If you're relying solely on plant-based sources for omega-3s, you're likely not getting enough EPA and DHA. Consider adding fish or algae-based supplements to your routine."

Ignoring Omega-6 Intake: Many people focus solely on increasing omega-3 intake without reducing omega-6 consumption. Dr. Joseph Hibbeln emphasizes, "Boosting omega-3 intake is important, but it won't be effective unless you also reduce your omega-6 consumption from processed foods and vegetable oils."

Choosing Low-Quality Supplements: Not all omega-3 supplements are created equal. Cheap fish oils may contain lower concentrations of EPA and DHA, and some may even be rancid. Dr. Andrew

Weil advises, "Invest in high-quality supplements that are properly stored and processed to avoid harmful oxidation."

By avoiding these common pitfalls and making informed choices about fats, you can significantly improve your omega-6 to omega-3 ratio and support long-term health.

the future of health – omega-3s and cutting-edge research

AS WE CONTINUE to unlock the health benefits of omega-3 fatty acids, new research emerges, suggesting even broader applications for these essential fats. From cancer prevention to mental health breakthroughs, and the role of omega-3s in personalized medicine, the future of health is deeply connected to our understanding of these vital nutrients. In this final chapter, we explore cutting-edge research that shows how omega-3s could shape the future of longevity and wellness.

Ongoing Research: Omega-3s in Cancer Prevention

Recent studies suggest that omega-3 fatty acids may play a role in reducing the risk of certain cancers, thanks to their anti-inflammatory properties. Chronic inflammation is known to contribute to cancer development by promoting cellular damage and tumor growth. Omega-3s, particularly EPA and DHA, may help mitigate this risk by lowering inflammation and influencing gene expression related to cancer progression.

A study published in 'Cancer Epidemiology, Biomarkers & Prevention' found that higher levels of omega-3s were associated with a reduced risk of breast cancer in postmenopausal women. Dr. José Russo, a cancer researcher notes, "Omega-3 fatty acids have shown promise in reducing the risk of hormone-related cancers like breast cancer by modulating estrogen metabolism and reducing inflammation."

Additionally, research from the 'Journal of Clinical Oncology' suggests that omega-3s may slow the growth of certain tumors by inhibiting angiogenesis—the process by which tumors develop new blood vessels. Dr. Edward Giovannucci, a leading cancer researcher adds, "Omega-3s appear to influence key biological processes involved in cancer development, making them a potential tool in both prevention and treatment."

While more large-scale studies are needed, the anti-inflammatory and tumor-suppressing effects of omega-3s could make them a valuable part of cancer prevention strategies in the future.

Mental Health Breakthroughs: Omega-3 in Treating Anxiety and Depression

Omega-3 fatty acids are increasingly recognized for their role in mental health, particularly in the treatment of anxiety and depression. The brain is rich in DHA, which supports neural function, neurotransmitter production, and inflammation regulation—all factors that influence mood and cognitive function. Growing evidence suggests that omega-3 supplementation can improve outcomes for individuals suffering from depression, anxiety, and other mental health disorders.

Dr. Joseph Hibbeln explains: "Omega-3s, particularly EPA, have been shown to reduce symptoms of depression by regulating the brain's inflammatory pathways and enhancing serotonin production." A meta-analysis published in 'Translational Psychiatry' found that omega-3 supplements, especially those rich in EPA, were effective in reducing depressive symptoms in individuals with major depressive disorder.

Moreover, a 2018 study in 'JAMA Network Open' highlighted the potential of omega-3s in treating anxiety, showing significant reductions in anxiety symptoms among participants who supplemented with high doses of EPA. Dr. Roel Mocking, a lead author on the study, emphasizes, "Omega-3 supplementation offers a promising adjunctive treatment for individuals with anxiety, particularly those who do not respond well to traditional treatments."

These findings suggest that omega-3s may become an integral part of mental health treatment protocols, offering a natural, non-pharmacological approach to managing mood disorders.

Future Trends: The Role of Omega-3 in Personalized Medicine

As the field of personalized medicine continues to evolve, omega-3s are likely to play a key role in tailoring health interventions to individual needs. Personalized medicine focuses on the unique genetic, environmental, and lifestyle factors that influence a person's health, allowing for more targeted and effective treatments. Omega-3s, with their broad range of benefits and their influence on gene expression, are perfectly suited to this approach.

A 2020 study published in 'Nutrients' found that individuals with certain genetic polymorphisms responded more favorably to omega-3 supplementation, particularly in terms of reducing inflammation and improving cardiovascular outcomes. Dr. Philip Calder, an expert in nutritional immunology, notes, "Personalized medicine is the future, and omega-3s offer a unique opportunity to tailor interventions based on genetic predispositions and metabolic profiles."

Additionally, omega-3 testing is becoming more common in functional medicine practices, allowing patients to adjust their omega-3 intake based on their specific needs and deficiencies. As Dr. Mark Hyman puts it, "By testing omega-3 levels and incorporating personalized recommendations, we can offer more precise and effective treatments for conditions ranging from heart disease to autoimmune disorders."

As research progresses, we may see omega-3s used in more sophisticated, individualized treatment plans that optimize health outcomes based on genetic and lifestyle factors.

What's Next: How Omega-3s Could Shape the Future of Longevity and Wellness

Omega-3 fatty acids have long been associated with longevity and wellness, thanks to their anti-inflammatory, heart-protective, and neuroprotective properties. As our understanding of these fats deepens, the potential for omega-3s to shape the future of aging and wellness is becoming clearer.

A groundbreaking study published in 'The American Journal of Clinical Nutrition' found that individuals with higher omega-3 levels had significantly lower risks of all-cause mortality. The study showed that those with the highest omega-3 concentrations lived an average of 2.2 years longer than those with lower levels. Dr. William Harris, co-author of the study, explains, "Higher omega-3 levels are associated with longevity, largely due to their ability to reduce inflammation, protect against cardiovascular disease, and preserve cognitive function."

The potential for omega-3s to promote healthy aging extends beyond heart and brain health. Omega-3s also support joint function, eye health, and immune regulation, all of which are crucial for maintaining vitality as we age. As Dr. Andrew Weil notes, "Omega-3s are one of the most powerful nutrients we have for promoting longevity. By incorporating them into a daily wellness routine, we can significantly improve the quality and length of our lives."

Looking ahead, continued research into omega-3s could reveal even more about their role in aging, disease prevention, and overall wellness, cementing their place as a cornerstone of healthy living for generations to come.

Fix Your Fats, Fuel Your Future

As we come to the end of this journey through the vital role omega-3 and omega-6 fatty acids play in our health, it's clear that these essential fats are more than just dietary components—they are the foundation of longevity, cellular function, and systemic health. By understanding the imbalance caused by our modern diet, and by making conscious efforts to fix our fats, we have the power to dramatically improve our health and the health of future generations.

Recap: The Omega Solution for Longevity, Cellular, and Systemic Health

Throughout this book, we've explored the profound impact that balancing omega-3 and omega-6 fatty acids can have on nearly every aspect of our well-being. Omega-3s, particularly EPA and DHA, are crucial for reducing inflammation, supporting heart and brain health, maintaining cellular integrity, and even promoting longevity. When these fats are in balance with omega-6, they work in harmony to regulate the body's inflammatory responses, protect against chronic diseases, and preserve cognitive function.

Dr. William Harris, has shown through numerous studies that higher omega-3 levels are associated with longer life expectancy and a lower risk of cardiovascular disease, cancer, and neurodegenerative disorders. This "Omega Solution" is not just about adding more omega-3s to your diet—it's about creating a balance that fosters long-term health and vitality.

Your Action Plan: Implementing the Omega-3 Solution in Daily Life

The path to reclaiming your health begins with simple but impactful changes to your diet and lifestyle. Here's how you can start implementing the Omega-3 Solution into your daily life:

Prioritize Omega-3-Rich Foods: Add fatty fish like salmon, sardines, and mackerel to your meals at least twice a week. Plant-based sources like flaxseeds, chia seeds, and walnuts can also help boost your omega-3 intake.

Reduce Omega-6 Consumption: Limit your intake of processed foods and oils high in omega-6, such as soybean, corn, and sunflower oils. Replace these with healthier options like olive oil, avocado oil, and grass-fed butter.

Consider Omega-3 Supplements: If it's difficult to meet your omega-3 needs through food alone, consider a high-quality fish oil or algal oil supplement that provides both EPA and DHA.

Track Your Progress: Use at-home omega-3 test kits to measure your omega-3 to omega-6 ratio and make adjustments as needed. Regular testing ensures that your efforts are moving you toward the right balance.

Dr. Mark Hyman advises, "The power to optimize your health is in your hands. By making these small but deliberate changes, you can reduce inflammation, improve your longevity, and support every system in your body."

The Journey to a Healthier, Longer Life Starts with the Right Fats

As we've learned, the fats we consume have a profound influence on our overall health. The journey to a healthier, longer life begins with making conscious choices about the types of fats we eat. By correcting the omega-3 to omega-6 imbalance, you're not only addressing inflammation, heart disease, and cognitive decline—you're setting yourself up for a vibrant, energized future.

This is not just a diet plan; it's a long-term investment in your health. As Dr. Andrew Weil notes, "The right fats are the foundation of well-being. They influence how we feel, how we age, and how we live. The earlier you start making changes, the more profound the benefits."

Sarah's Health Legacy: A Story of Reclamation and Generational Impact

As we reflect on Sarah's journey, it's clear that the changes she made weren't just about addressing her immediate health concerns—they were about reclaiming her future. By focusing on correcting her fats and addressing the omega-3 to omega-6 imbalance, Sarah was able to reverse the chronic issues that had plagued her for years. But the impact didn't stop with her.

Through her new understanding of nutrition, Sarah has equipped her children with the knowledge and habits to make healthier choices.

This health legacy won't just affect her children; it will ripple through three or four generations of her family, creating a foundation of wellness that will benefit her grandchildren and beyond.

Dr. Joseph Mercola often speaks about the generational impact of health decisions, saying, "When we make health-conscious choices, we're not just improving our own lives—we're setting an example for future generations. The decisions you make today could prevent chronic disease for your children and grandchildren."

Sarah's story is a reminder that health is a lifelong journey, but it's also a gift that can be passed down. By fixing her fats, Sarah isn't just reclaiming her own health—she's creating a legacy of wellness that will pay dividends for generations to come.

In the end, the journey to optimal health starts with one simple step: fixing your fats and fueling your future.

Sarah's 100+Living Plan consisted of more than just her nutritional choices although this is the pillar we focused on in this book. As I hinted in the section that discussed Saraha's IBS diagnosis, her neurology was compromised as well. Please use the resources at the end of this book to reach out to a doctor in your area that is certified and experienced in diagnosing adult spinal deformity, and I wish you great success in your health recovery.

a request for your honest feedback

Now that you are finished my book I'd like to invite you to share your thoughts and experiences by leaving an honest review on Amazon. Your feedback is not only important to me but also instrumental in enhancing the overall quality of this book. I am committed to delivering content that goes above and beyond your expectations, and your insights play a crucial role in achieving this.

Reviews not only help prospective readers make informed decisions but also provide me with an opportunity to address any areas that may need further clarification or expansion.

Your reviews enable me to refine the content, fill any gaps that may exist, and ensure that the information presented is accessible and applicable to a wide audience.

My commitment to you is to deliver more value than you expect from this book. Your feedback will not only help shape the future editions but also contribute to the creation of a community dedicated to positive change and holistic well-being.

Thank you again for investing your time with my book, I look forward to hearing your thoughts and insights. Together, we can make a difference in the lives of many.

Wishing you health and happiness,

Dr. J

resources to take what you have read to a higher level

As a doctor who has dedicated his career to a life of learning, changing and adapting I want to introduce you to some incredible resources that may help you in your journey to restore your sleep and reclaim your health. The first is a world wide doctor directory of CBP certified doctors. Ideally you want to find an advanced certified CBP doctor but I admit, we are few and far between. Check out this website to see if there is an advanced certified CBP office near you, or at least a doctor who has begun their training with a basic certification.

https://idealspine.com/directory/

My clinic website is also a great resource, and I am adding content to my blog section each month. You can find my clinic website here. Check out the blog section. . .

https://lighthousehealth.ca/

If you have any questions about what you have read and want to reach out to me directly for input, support or some of my online courses like Re-Position our posture restoration course, you can email me directly at. . .

drj@lighthousehealth.ca

My You Tube channel has content that supports what we have talked about in this book, you can access it free here at the link below. . . . or search Graham Jenkins @LighthouseKelowna on You Tube
https://www.youtube.com/channel/
UCOVX9MFEsaid5g7z73CITkA

And finally, the same place you found this book, Amazon, will give you access to my 100+Living Series of books. I trust that I've given you the encouragement to change your lifestyle and adopt the strategies that have propelled my patients to their best health with The 100+Living Plan.

Consult with a Trusted Health Practitioner

As with all health advice that you read in a book or encounter online, it's crucial that you consult with a healthcare practitioner you know and trust before making any significant changes to your health routines.

While I can share expert quotes and suggestions, I am not your personal doctor, and there are unique nuances in your health history and current condition that I cannot know through the pages of a book.It is always important to approach health changes with caution, and a trusted health professional can guide you through the specifics of what is best for your body and your circumstances. If you do not currently have a healthcare provider you trust, please refer to the resource section of this book, where I have recommended experienced doctors who may be able to help.

Please remember, the content in the 100+Living series, including this book, is for informational purposes only. It is not intended to replace personalized health care advice, and any health strategies discussed should not be implemented without the support and full knowledge of a trusted health professional.

In health,
Dr. J